NO MORE MEDS

Bella,
much love & many Blessings!
Enjoy!
CW

DR. CORINNE E. WEAVER, DC

Unless otherwise indicated, all Scripture quotations marked NIV are taken from the Holy Bible, New International Version.

NO MORE MEDS

ISBN-13: 978-1545521687

ISBN 10: 1545521689

Dr. Corinne E. Weaver, DC

14015-D East Independence Blvd.

Indian Trail, NC 28079

Websites:

www.DrCorinneWeaver.com

www.GetWellNC.com

www.CharlotteADDhelp.com

www.DrWeaversWater.com

www.PhysicalBreathing.com

www.DrCorinne.tv

www.NoMoreMedsMovement.com

DISCLAIMER

The educational information and guidelines contained in this book are based upon the research and the personal and professional experiences of the author. They are not intended as a substitute for consultation with your health care provider. This information is for educational purposes only and has not been evaluated by the Food and Drug Administration. These products and the information are not intended to diagnose, treat, cure, or prevent disease.

DISCLOSURE ABOUT CASE STUDIES IN THIS BOOK

I have included some case studies from my own practice in this book. These specific case studies were intentionally chosen to help you relate to actual patients and their lives. I shared this book with several of my patients before its release, and they said that the case study stories gave them hope when there was none. Even though the concepts presented in the case studies are not guaranteed to help everyone, we must have hope when we are working on improving our health! I hope these stories motivate you and provide positive energy to assist you on your journey. To ensure individuals' privacy, however, I have changed some of the names in the stories.

Now, it is time to follow the yellow brick road…

DEDICATION

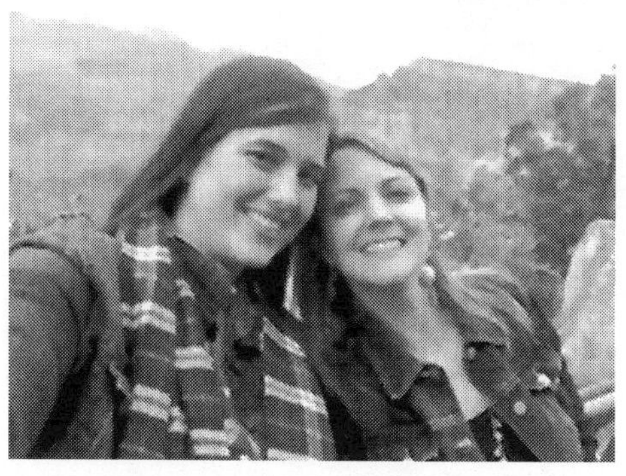

I dedicate this book to my wonderful friend Stephanie, who is married and has four beautiful children. Thanks for allowing me to be a part of your family. You always have been there for me since the day we met in 1997 when we were 18 and attending Camp Quest (a Christian camp that changed our lives forever). I am blessed to have you as a friend in Christ and a prayer warrior who dances her heart out for what is right!

I wrote this book to help parents who are overwhelmed by the daily stress they experience because they have sick and oversensitive kids.

I also dedicate this book to my mom, who did not know how to take care of herself when I was a sick kid—instead, she let her own health slip away (just as I didn't know how to take care of myself when I was taking care of her). I was very sick, and as I was trying to learn how to get better, I got sicker and sicker because of stress. I didn't realize how sick I was until my mom was gone and I was 60 pounds overweight and exhausted. I desperately needed help. Fortunately, I finally found solutions, and now I want to share those solutions with you.

How many moms go through the same thing?

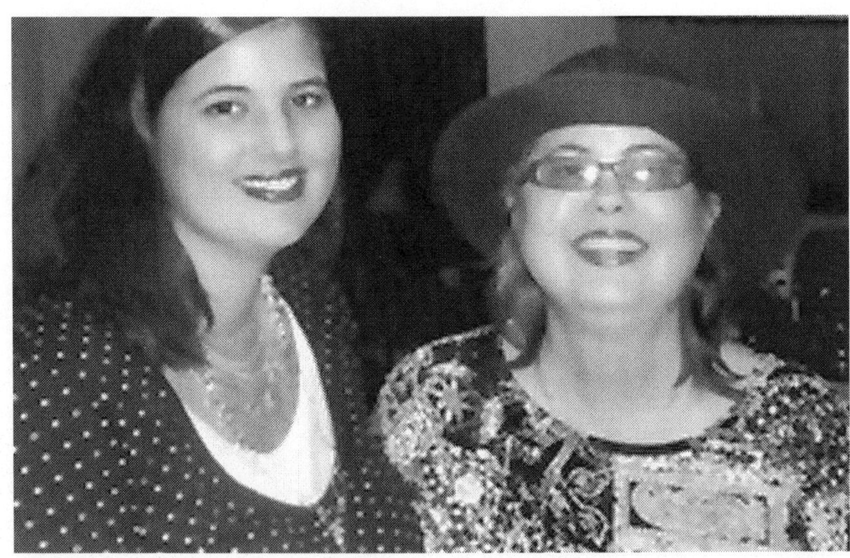

ADVANCE PRAISE

"All parents want their children to be healthy and happy, and Dr. Weaver has plenty of advice to help parents help their kids, from providing tips about natural remedies and relaxation exercises to explaining how to choose better foods for the entire family. This is a useful book for parents no matter how old their children are--lots here for adults, too!"

- Lisa Howard,
Author of Healthier Gluten-Free and The Big Book of Healthy Cooking Oils

"As a mom and a doctor, Dr. Corinne Weaver has a special love for children and to see all children grow up healthy. Her passion, heart, and knowledge come through powerfully in the pages of this book.

Regardless of your knowledge level, *No More Meds* provides a wealth of information, both for the person wanting to start a healthy lifestyle and for the established health professional.

This is especially a must-read book for parents who desire to start their families on a life path free of drugs and full of health.

Dr. Weaver's life journey makes her uniquely qualified to offer insight and expert advice in the ways of natural health."

- Dr. Michael Anderson, DC

Refreshing to see and hear the basic concepts of health portrayed in a way that's so easily understood. Great job, Dr. Corinne!

- Dr. Greg Melvin, DC and Board Certified Clinical Thermologist

ACKNOWLEDGMENTS

I want to thank first my husband, Scott, who has been by my side during every step of our journey. His constant encouragement has made me realize I can do all things through Christ, who strengthens me. Scott always goes above and beyond his call of duty, and I am forever his Sunny Delight. Also, thanks to my beautiful kids, whose minds impress me every day. It's because of your brains that I live on to share my brain.

Thanks, Dad, for always telling me to go after my dreams and reach for the stars.

Thanks to my grandfather, who also wrote a book (his book is called *Furrow in the Clouds*). His positive thinking and fight to survive made me who I am today. I am so honored to be his granddaughter.

I want to thank my Uncle John, who inspired me to learn about natural healing and helped me see how I can inspire others.

To all the parents who have trusted me to take care of their sick kids over the years.

Thanks to my wonderful team: Dr. Lisa Plesa, Marie Green, Adora Zachary, Ann Berryman, and Gil Meijer.

On your pathway to wellness, remember that healing comes from the inside. Enjoy your journey!

Dr. Corinne E. Weaver, DC
March 2017

TABLE OF CONTENTS

FOREWORD

My healing journey never stops. I am grateful for every day. From living with cancer, I know the value of keeping myself mentally and physically balanced and healthy.

I know the importance of learning those good habits from an early age. When I was a child I wish that I had a Doctor like Dr. Corinne Weaver. Her special love for children and her passion to see them all grow up healthy is inspiring. She understands that our individual life experiences make us each unique.

Dr. Weaver's book shows us that we have a healthcare crisis that is negatively affecting our kid's immune systems and brain sensitivities. The strategies she provides will help you and your child strengthen your immune systems and calm your nerves.

We live in a stressful world, so it's good to have access to Dr. Corinne's Stress-Free System. It's important that children and their parents have effective and meaningful communication. Effective communication starts with listening not only with your ears but with your heart and being mindful of the nonverbal communication coming from your child.

Follow Dr. Corinne's breathing exercises and help create a deeper more intimate relationship with your children.

Olivia Newton-John, OBE, OA
Singer and Actress

INTRODUCTION

"Children are the world's most valuable resource and its best hope for the future." – John F. Kennedy

Have you ever searched the internet for answers to these questions or asked your doctor any of them?

- Why is my kid sick all the time?
- Why is my kid crying over every little thing?
- Why does my kid only eat pancakes and is so picky?
- What's wrong with my child's personality?
- Why is my kid mad and angry over the little things?
- Why is my kid so sensitive to smells, sounds, and lights?
- I remember when my kid was healthy until this [a physical, chemical, and/or emotional trauma] happened. Can I go back?

As parents, we all want our kids to be safe and healthy. In this book, I will be teaching you how to keep your kids healthy so that they don't need more meds.

What keeps us healthy? It's simple: a strong immune system!! So then here are more questions: how do we help our children have strong immune systems? As parents, are we doing an excellent job of building our children's immune systems?

Unfortunately, the answer to that last question is no. If kids in America were healthy, I wouldn't be writing this book. It makes me so sad to see little kids suffering from allergies, asthma, acid reflux, cognitive and behavioral disorders like ADD/ADHD, insomnia, autoimmune conditions, seizures, heavy metal toxicity, and developmental delays. The proof is in the statistical pudding: 25.5 million children under the age of 18 are taken to the ER each year.

What are the top ten most common reasons for ER visits (according to U.S. News & World Report)?

1. Injuries and poisoning
2. Respiratory disorders like asthma
3. Nervous system disorders like sports-related concussions and seizures
4. Infections and parasitic diseases
5. Digestive disorders
6. Skin disorders
7. Mental and behavioral health conditions such as depression
8. Musculoskeletal disorders like sprains
9. Genitourinary disorders like a urinary tract infection
10. Endocrine disorders like diabetes

When I look at the top ten list, I wonder how we as parents can keep our kids from constantly going to the ER like I did when I was growing up. Where are all of these problems coming from?

The answers came to me when I got a call last year from my best friend who was dealing with her sick kid. I wanted to help as much as I could, just like I have helped thousands of kids over my past 13 years as a wellness practitioner. I am an upper cervical chiropractor who lives a drug-free and pro-wellness lifestyle, and I love helping children heal naturally from allergies, asthma, ADD/ADHD, anxiety, and autism. As I was educating my friend about what to do, I realized there was so much to teach her about how to raise healthy kids. She knew my kids were healthy and have never needed any medications, but she didn't know what steps to take for her own child. She was sick of dealing with the medical system and not getting answers from her child's doctor.

It hit me: I had to write this book for her so that I could help her kids stay healthy. Thus, this journey began. As a doctor who was a sick kid myself and as a mom of a child with learning disabilities, I can relate to kids and to parents.

I want you as parents to understand the connections between the immune system and the brain. I want you to understand why your kid's immune system is weak and why their brain is not working right. I want you to know what foods are healing for the immune system and how to calm your and your kid's nerves. I want you to know what diagnostic tests and therapies are the best to do and why. There is hope. You as the parent can get help to help your child's body and brain heal.

My heart's desire with this book is to bring you peace by outlining what to do when your child's health is failing. Ideally, I would like for you to read this book before your child's health is bad—prevention is key!—but sadly, most parents won't make the time to learn about health issues and make substantial life changes until their child's health is failing.

Let's hope you got this book from a friend who cares about you and your child; let's hope you have just slightly started to head down the wrong path. Let me take you down the yellow brick road just long enough for you to realize that the answers are within you—you just need to see the Emerald City to get to them.

God promises that if we pursue Him, He will not only provide for our needs (Matthew 6:33), but He will give us our desires as well (Psalm 37:4-5).

And as the lyrics of "Somewhere Over the Rainbow" say, "Somewhere over the rainbow, skies are blue and the dreams that you dare to dream really do come true."

I absolutely love what I do, and I am excited to get this great information out to all of you.

I pray my second book speaks to you and you can wake up each morning with a purpose. What I do every day is a calling, and I give God the glory for allowing his gifts to work through me. I do believe in miracles, because I get to see them every day!!!!

As my aunt Olivia Newton-John would sing, "NOT GONNA GIVE IN TO IT!" and "Sometimes there is a miracle just beyond the pain, and you can see the rainbow in the rain…LIV ON!!!"

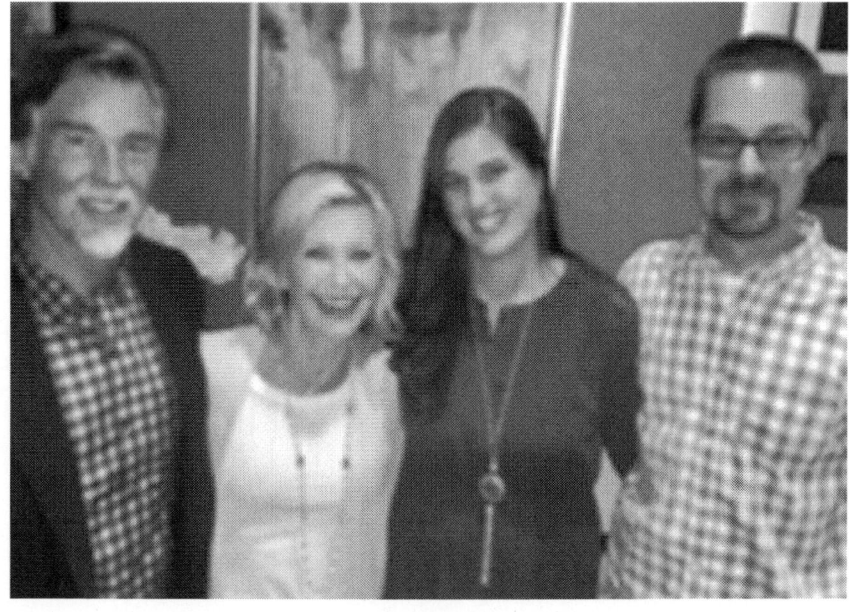

Chapter 1

DO WE HAVE A HEALTHCARE CRISIS?

My Story

It was a beautiful, hot 4th of July afternoon—a perfect day to swim at the neighborhood pool with my best friend. I loved to swim, and being 10 years old, I was very good at it. After swimming, we decided to go get some lunch at home, so we left the pool and I jumped on the brand-new pink bicycle I had gotten for Christmas. As I was riding along, a horsefly landed on my shoulder. I reached over to knock it off, and *boom!* Next thing I knew, I was flying over my handlebars.

I woke up and realized I was in a hospital. My front tooth was gone and I couldn't breathe. That day changed my health forever: I needed twenty stitches on my bottom lip and had to get my tooth capped, so I could hardly eat anything for about a month. The only thing I did was lay on the couch, drink milkshakes, and look at a TV for the rest the summer. When my mouth healed, I thought everything was going to get better, but it didn't. I became a "hypersensitive child."

What I mean by this is that every little thing seemed to bother my breathing, and I became allergic to my surroundings. The doctors my parents took me to never looked at my spine as causing any of the symptoms I was having—they just treated my symptoms with medication. My journey of taking medicine began.

I was given breathing machines and an inhaler; my life became living on breathing machines twice a day and having an inhaler in my pocket that was always at my beck and call.

My breathing was so bad my parents had to take me to an allergy specialist to figure out what I was allergic to that could be causing my asthma attacks. They found out I was allergic to everything outside: grass, weeds, trees, mold, flowers, mildew. And I was allergic to dust and cats, too.

My parents had to get rid of our cats, carpets, stuffed animals, and lots more. We had to stop going to our old church because it was moldy and I had an asthma attack every time we went. My grandmother had to remove all her flowers and potpourri whenever we went over to her house.

I was always living on the edge, not knowing when I would have another asthma attack. It was so scary being a kid who was constantly struggling to breathe. I thought there was no end in sight to my misery—my nervous system was extremely overreactive and making my body horribly oversensitive. I love my parents and knew that they were doing everything they knew to do to get me better, but the only solutions the doctors had to offer were more drugs. What was all of this costing my parents? Even though insurance paid for some of my ER and doctor visits, my medical issues were still costing my parents hundreds of dollars a month and not offering any real solutions. Now, if my parents had paid thousands of dollars and I was getting better, they would have never complained. But the reality was all the money they spent was just covering up my symptoms and never getting down to the root cause of the problem.

I suffered from my disease for years—in fact, I experienced exactly 11 years of surgeries, pain, and poor health. If only my parents had met a doctor like the one I've become, that doctor could have saved them thousands of dollars and my quality of life!!

The Way Modern Healthcare Works

Imagine if the healthcare system cared about patients and looked deeper into their problems to come up with top-quality solutions instead of just masking symptoms. My vision is to have doctors develop better relationships with their patients/clients and take the time to truly find solutions that make a difference in their quality of life. I want the healthcare system to have doctors who work together for the good of the patients/clients and not have to solely depend on the treatments and services that insurance allows.

Recently, I was at Harvard and talking to a plastic surgeon who had practiced medicine for 30 years. He was saying that for every breast cancer patient he sees, he must spend about 5-6 hours compiling notes for the insurance companies to get them to pay for the treatments; even then, he said, insurance still fights against paying. Because of insurance paperwork, he said, he doesn't have time to discuss quality-of-care issues. He said his patients were now experiencing more complications because of this.

He ended the conversion by saying that if something doesn't change, he was advising medical students to choose another profession because of the stress load that comes along with being a doctor. He'll be retiring next year, he said, and the smile on his face told me how excited he was to stop having to deal with the insurance madness. Of course, he hopes something will change with patient care, but he said he doesn't see changes happening anytime soon.

Your Child's Health

Take a moment to consider what you know about your child. You may not realize to what extent sickness can affect your child and therefore the entire family. You might be under the impression that your child is unruly or impossible to keep in line when the truth is that every child's brain and body is unique and has unique needs.

I believe that stress is a big trigger for people who are sick, whether they're children or adults. If your child is sick and/or is having a meltdown, it is critical that you try very hard not to react to the action itself. Instead, try to identify the source of the stress and then reduce or eliminate it so then you can redirect your child's attention and get them back on track.

If you cannot identify what is causing or triggering the sickness, it can be very frustrating. You may want to know what else you can do to help your child, such as ways to strengthen your child's immune system and coping skills so they can handle stress better and have fewer meltdowns. I can provide you with ways to improve these situations, because yes, there is hope!

In my practice, we use amazing methods (which I will be discussing later on in the book) to strengthen your child's immune system and heal their brain and body functions with remarkable success. We see impressive results with this type of brain-based therapy. Kids with ADD and/or ADHD, anxiety, allergies, asthma, autism, and autoimmune conditions—to name just a few "A" diagnoses—have very sensitive systems. They can get overwhelmed very easily, and they may have trouble coping with stress or too much information or activity at once. Their nervous systems are quite sensitive, and you may notice that they are "picky" when it comes to the five senses.

What do I mean by sensitivity to senses? These children may reject certain foods or want to eat only a few foods. They may react to loud noises, bright lights, or strong odors. They may be very sensitive to certain textures. Clothing which feels fine to you might feel incredibly uncomfortable or itchy to them. Daily life can feel like a barrage or an assault on their senses.

Using our established healing methods, we can help children (and adults, too) who have these conditions process unpleasant stimuli more easily. By giving them coping mechanisms, strengthening their skills, and building their immune systems, we are helping them lead lives that are more positive and fulfilling.

In addition to focusing on sources of stresses and triggers, we also pay attention to your child's daily diet: we want to know if your child is getting enough nutrients, vitamins, minerals, and even enough calories. Many people—not just those with ADD and/or ADHD, anxiety, allergies, asthma, autism, and autoimmune disorders—respond to situations poorly and have fewer coping skills when they are just plain hungry or thirsty. We are sure you will agree that a properly nourished and hydrated person is better equipped to handle problems or stress! Drinking only water (1 quart per 50 pounds of body weight per day) is ideal. You can go to www.drweaverswater.com to find out which water filter I love best, namely the kind that removes fluoride, which is a neurotoxin. I encourage parents to make sure they are taking care of their own needs, too, so they can better handle stress and be the best parent for their child.

In addition to analyzing the nutrition a child is or is not getting, we look at potential food allergies or food sensitivities the child may have. We know that having an allergic reaction to food makes a person feel awful. Now imagine having a slightly less severe food allergy. It might not be life-threatening, but it can still make a person feel unwell. It's understandable that a person—child or adult—with an unknown food allergy might feel stressed. This stress can lead to behavioral issues and sickness.

Our attention to detail makes all the difference! When it comes to you or your loved one who has these hypersensitivities, we want to find the root cause of the condition. We want to work with you to help your children realize their potential. We want to help identify any challenges they have and strengthen their coping skills so that when they face challenges and stresses, they can move past them and thrive. And we want to do all of this without resorting to drug interventions.

Our Drug Culture

Why in America do we depend on so many drugs to survive? We are taught in school to "Say no to drugs!", but when I was a kid, I also knew I had to take drugs for the rest of my life to survive. I was a very confused kid!!

Now that it is 2017, you would think America's drug crisis would be better, but it isn't. I hate to say this, but actually our drug crisis has gotten worse each year. Why do we think if we take this or that magical pill all our problems will go away? Have we been brainwashed? After all, the US consumes far more painkillers than any other country in the world.

What are we so scared of? Fear itself. The whole medical system is based on fear. Simply put, doctors began to fill out a record number of prescriptions for drugs to treat patients' conditions. That led to people getting hooked on painkillers and then moving over to using illegal drugs such as heroin when they were eventually unable to keep getting their prescriptions for painkillers. More recently, people have begun using fentanyl, an opioid that's even more potent and cheaper than heroin. The result is more deaths. When are we going to wake up and realize that drugs are not the answer?

For me, it took me continually getting sicker to realize that the medicine cabinet did not have the answers I needed.

Why do we consume so many drugs? Because we trust our doctors and they write drug prescriptions for us. Starting in the 1980s and 90s, doctors were under pressure to take pain more seriously. There were (and still are) some good reasons for that: according to a 2011 report from the Institute of Medicine, about 100 million Americans still suffer from chronic pain.

The result of the prescription trend was that in 2012, US doctors wrote 259 million prescriptions for painkillers, enough to give a bottle of pills to every adult in the country. And these pills didn't just end up in patients' hands—they were shared among friends and family, they landed in the hands of teens who rummaged through their parents' medicine cabinets, and so on. This stat just makes me want to add my sad emoji face. We are raising our kids to think that if something hurts, they should just take a pill.

One of the undeniable contributors to the painkiller epidemic is drug companies. Drug companies pitched newer products like OxyContin as the big medical solution. The marketing was extremely misleading, often presenting these drugs as safer and more effective than other painkillers on the market…but then we found out that these drugs were in fact extremely addictive and dangerous. After all, if these drugs did work, why do American still report higher levels of chronic pain? Again, I say that drugs are not the answer.

There's simply no good scientific evidence that painkillers can treat long-term pain, because patients grow tolerant of the painkilling effects. There is, however, plenty of evidence that prolonged use can result in very bad complications, including higher risks of addiction, overdose, and death. That should scare us.

After long-term use, some patients who try to stop taking painkillers will feel a sudden surge of pain. They'll likely think the pain they're feeling is their chronic pain coming back in full force now that the painkillers are gone. The truth, however, is that the opioids had already likely stopped working on the original chronic pain due to the patient's ever-increasing tolerance—

that sudden surge of pain is an entirely new pain from drug-dependence withdrawal, not the original chronic pain.

There's also evidence that opioids can make pain worse. Opioids might make people more sensitive to pain and weaken the bones, for one thing. Opioids also might prompt people to do things that expose them to greater injury, which of course leads to far more pain—for example, because the patient feels no pain, he or she might do more housework than usual, leading to more long-term damage because the patient is not resting. I come across this scenario every day in my practice.

According to the April 2016 issue of *Fortune*, US drug spending hit a record high again: per the IMS Institute for Healthcare Informatics, hospitals and pharmacies spent $424.8 billion on drugs.

So if drugs aren't the answer to healing the body, what is?

There are alternative therapies that can be very beneficial, although these can involve more work, education, and money on the patient's part compared to just taking a pill (we will discuss these therapies later in the book).

Here are some alarming stats on people who have certain conditions.

- 322 million people of all ages suffer from depression (1).
- 264 million adults suffer from anxiety (1).
- 6.4 million children in America have ADHD; the yearly cost of this is $42.5 billion (2).
- 28 million Americans suffer from migraines, according to the National Headache Foundation.
- 1 in 3 adults don't get enough sleep, according to a CDC newsroom release in February 2016.

Our country needs to devise solutions for how to get people to stop using drugs. If a patient must have a drug, we need to know how to make their drug use less deadly and dangerous (3).

The reality is that at some level, some patients who are struggling with chronic health issues may just have to learn to find alternative therapies and realize that the answer isn't in a pill.

Alternative Therapies Do Work

When I was a kid, my amazing Uncle John (who would spend time in the Amazon jungle in South America learning about Amazon herbs) would come to town and make me some fresh herbal tea. I would breathe in that tea with a kitchen towel draped over my head, and my lungs would open and alleviate my most severe breathing symptoms. Even as a small kid, I knew I liked breathing in that tea much better than using the nasty steroid breathing machine I had. The taste of the roots and barks was disgusting, true, but I would breath in their tea anyway, because after I did, I felt better. I knew something in those herbs he gave me was powerful.

Uncle John gave me the first hope that I could get off the breathing machines and drugs I was taking, but still, as the years went by, my asthma and allergies got worse with all of the added drugs and shots I was taking. Then, while visiting my Uncle one summer, everything became clear. He had just been in a car accident and had fractured his back. As he was lying on the couch in tons of pain, I felt the need to help him. He did not take painkillers—he only used natural remedies to help heal his body. He asked me to apply recovery herbs to his back and work on aligning the energy in his spine. I had no idea what I was doing, but I nonetheless felt empowered to help him. After I worked on him for about an hour, he woke up and said he felt the best he had felt since the accident. He looked at me and said, "You have healing hands."

I felt empowered to help others feel better with my healing hands, a feeling that was reinforced when Uncle John introduced me to chiropractic principles. I fell in love with the philosophy of chiropractic care!! Our bodies have the power to heal from the inside—the power that made the body can heal the body. The nervous system runs the whole body, and if there is no interference with brain-to-body communication, the body can operate at its optimum.

As I grew older, I developed a strong relationship with God. At a summer Christian camp called Camp Quest, I prayed and asked, "Lord, what do you want me to be when I grow up?" I heard the word loud and clear in my mind: "Chiropractor!" Part of our job is to listen well to the Word of God and the Spirit of God. We are good at talking to God, but we aren't good at listening to God. From that day on, I dedicated my life to help others with their healing, and now I hope to bring healing to you through my words in this book.

During my eight years of studying the nervous, immune, and hormonal systems, I came to understand that the physical stress of my bike accident had caused my health to take a bad turn and the doctors I saw to make mistakes. That said, please know that I didn't write this book to bash medical professionals—in fact, I am very thankful that they could handle the severe symptoms I was having when I was a kid. I am just saying that I wish doctors would look more deeply into the root causes of a problem instead of just masking its symptoms.

If a doctor would've taken the time to look and see that my symptoms started after the bike accident and to see that the physical head trauma had started a series of sickness in my body, that doctor could have reached out to another doctor to see if that physical head trauma was causing breathing issues for me. I just needed a doctor to get my head on straight, pun intended!!

But that accident was not a coincidence: it was my destiny to learn how to heal my body so I could help thousands of others do the same. I feel so blessed that God led me to figure out how to heal myself, and I want to share these amazing healing secrets with you, too, so that you can also heal.

I married my high school sweetheart at the early age of 20 and went to college to study the philosophy of how our body has the power to heal from inside. I was so excited to learn this was possible! While in chiropractic school, I received regular chiropractic care, specifically upper cervical care. All of my asthma/allergy symptoms disappeared within a year—I threw all my drugs away and have not had to rely on them ever again, and it's been over 16 years now.

I went on to finish my schooling and then opened my practice in 2004. I have three wonderful children; I gave birth to them all naturally at home and none of them have ever had *any* drugs. I love helping women have natural childbirths and educating parents on how to raise healthy children naturally. This is my passion: helping kids be kids and enjoy lives free from chronic illness.

With brain dysfunction increasing (especially in children), we need more doctors who are trained in brain restoration. In this book, I will show you several lifestyle, diet, and non-drug approaches that can help your child regain their immune system and brain health while simultaneously experiencing fewer side effects than they would with conventional medications. The main goals of these lifestyle-based efforts are to reduce inflammation in their body and brain and restore their brain-to-body functions.

I Phil. 3:12

Not that I have already obtained all this, or have already arrived at my goal, but I press on to take hold of that for which Christ Jesus took hold of me.

Chapter 2

WHAT THREE STEPS CAN YOU TAKE TODAY TO IMPROVE YOUR CHILD'S MOOD?

Why I am starting out my book with improving your child's mood? Well, as a kid who was sick all the time and as a frustrated parent with a sick kid, I know that it's hard to be happy. We seem to always concentrate on the problems and not the solutions. I want you to be able to reread this chapter many times and remind your kid of these simple steps they can use to improve their mood so that they don't go mentally insane while dealing with their sickness. Twelve years ago, my mom was diagnosed with Stage 5 glioblastoma brain cancer and was given three months to live. Even though we eventually did lose her to cancer, she was able to live three years instead of three months. During that challenging time, I learned a lot about how to improve my mood. I will be sharing those methods with you as well as some stories of patients I have seen over the last 13 years of practice.

I hope these stories will speak to your heart and motivate you to *smile* more. According to an article, called "Why faking a smile is a good thing" in *Forbes* magazine on February 26, 2013, "Smilers exhibited lower heart rate levels after completing a stressful task compared to subjects who assumed a neutral expression."

The question I want you to ask your child right now is this: "Can you do these three steps today?"

1. Breathe! Our kids are not taking the time to take deep breaths; kids are always on the go-go-go. I understand. I have three kids and am constantly seeing them run here and there. The good thing is about this step is that you don't have to take a lot of time to breathe—all you need is a pair of lungs and a few minutes a day.

You can train your kids to take deep belly breaths throughout the day. The more your kid takes deep breaths, the more natural that kind of deep, easy breathing becomes. When your kids have better control of their breathing, they can lower their blood pressure and help their bodies de-stress. Bear in mind that when children are under a lot of stress, it is very hard for them to control their breath, so practice deep breathing now in order for your kids to have better control when stress hits.

Later in the book, I will teach you how you can do physical breathing any time and any place with your child. When my mom had cancer, every time I was with her, we took deep breaths together. Taking deep breaths together with your child helps you both relax—the brain will tell the body it's in a safe place.

2. Give your children a gratitude journal and have them listen to positive, uplifting music while they write down things they are thankful for. My all-time favorite song is "Grace and Gratitude" by Olivia Newton-John. (Olivia would come to my mom's log cabin and massage her feet while singing this song.) The act of expressing

gratitude can be so healing for your child's soul! We all have something to be thankful for, especially your child—they just need to be aware of it. My children love their gratitude journals. Mostly, they're full of beautiful images they create. (Even though my mom had been diagnosed with the most horrible brain cancer, she wrote in a gratitude journal almost every day, too.) Helping your child see the good in life can bring healing to the brain-and-body connection and offer hope to their little soul.

I thought I was always going to need my meds to survive daily life because that was what I always heard, but when a doctor told me "Your body can heal itself and you don't need these meds anymore," there was something inside me that started to believe this. My whole belief system had to change for me to be healed. I woke up and saw a new light.

3. Smile! My mom smiled all the time, and everyone who knew her knew her smile and her loud laugh. I smile a lot, too—in a card my mom made me in 2005, she wrote "I see God in your smile." My smile brought her joy! Amazing how a simple smile can change your attitude in life. She also knew how much I love dolphins and sand dollars, so she drew them on the card that I am sharing below. Every time I go to the beach and see dolphins and find sand dollars, it is like she is sending them my way to smile at me!!

Sand dollars represent peace, and peace is what I want you to receive from reading this. A few years ago, a patient shared the inside of a sand dollar with me. She told me that if I were to break open the sand dollar, five doves would appear. These doves are awaiting you, ready to spread good will and peace. God is everywhere and desires to heal you from the inside.

Dear Corinne, Scott, Noah,

I am so truly blessed to have such a wonderful family. We will get thru this with God's strength. I see God in your smile. I cherish our days together. I miss Noah alot, the times on Mon + Tues. I am so proud of you and Scott with what all you have done. I pray each day to listen wholeheartedly to God. He sent you to us as our Earthbound Angel. I can't wait to see Noah in his play. He is so precious. Check on me and Dad when you get time. It's been so hard on Dad. We need alot of faith.

We love you guys so much—

Mom + Dad

2005

Thank you so much for adjusting me

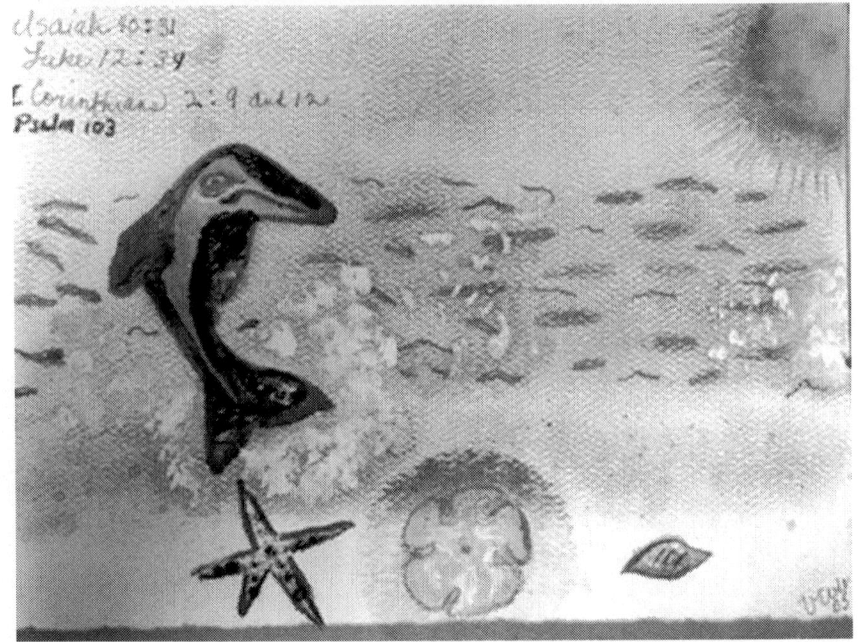

In *Elf*, a movie that my kids love to watch all year long, Will Ferrell is asked why he's smiling, and he responds by saying, "Smiling is my favorite!!"

Smiling lowers your heart rate and makes you feel happy inside. Just like the song from *Annie* says, "You are never fully dressed without a smile."

Back to expressing gratitude. Every day this week, I want to encourage you and your child to write down at least seven things you are grateful for. (You can write down more if you want, of course.) The diary my mom and I shared is so precious to me. She was thankful for her cancer because it brought us closer together, and memories of us writing in her journal are truly the best. Take this time to pray for your child, be alone with your thoughts, listen, let everything external in the world go, and be at peace. "Be still, know that I am God." Psalm 46:10

1.____

2.____

3.____

4.____

5.____

6.____

7.____

Make this a fun activity! If you want to make journaling your ritual, I'll send you a free gratitude journal. You will love it!!

All you need to do is email me at dr@drcorinneweaver.com. We'll schedule a call to talk about your child's health goals, and at the end of the call, remind me to send you your gratitude journal. I'll put one in the mail to you for free.

Now that we know the three steps we can take to improve our children's mood, here is what you should do to keep your child's S-T-R-E-S-S low so that their brain and body can function better and your child can heal.

DR. CORINNE'S **S-T-R-E-S-S FREE** SYSTEM

S-chedule time to learn why my kid is sick

T-esting and therapies

R-elax and release

E-ssential oils

S-upplements and herbs

S-leep

Chapter 3

S-CHEDULE TIME TO LEARN WHY MY KID IS SICK

The first letter of my S-T-R-E-S-S Free System is "S" for *"S-chedule time to learn why my kid is sick."*

First, let's define what health is: it is a state of optimal physical, emotional, and spiritual well-being. Health is not merely the absence of disease or "feeling good."

Four Types of Stress

1. Physical Stress

Physical stress is a physical trauma that causes our brain not to function properly (my bike accident was a physical stress). Accidents happen—they're part of a kid's life. What most people do not understand, however, is that even the smallest trauma (i.e., a stubbed toe) can send the body into a downward spiral. Unfortunately, most of the time, this dis-ease will not develop into symptoms until you have already forgotten about that little "trauma." The American Pediatrics Association estimates that the average child falls 5,000 times as they learn to walk! And did you know that 8 out of 10 newborns are born with an atlas subluxation? The trauma of birth and the connection to neck strain was the subject of an extensive research project by two German medical physicians. Dr. Guttman concluded that about 80% of all children are not in autonomic balance of the autonomic nervous system and may have a subluxation (4). A subluxation means they have interference within the brain-to-body communication that is taking place in their central nervous system (CNS). His colleague, Dr. Frymann examined a random group of 1250 babies, 5 days posterior partum. Manual examination revealed cervical strain in 95% of this group (4). Therefore, it is vital to have your child checked by an upper cervical doctor who can remove the subluxation and restore normal nerve system function and greater health.

2. Chemical Stress

We wake up in the morning and use heavily (and artificially) scented shampoos and soaps. Our teenagers put on deodorant that contains aluminum, which clogs up their lymphatic system. We as parents use dryer sheets with artificial scents to make our clothes smell good. All of these chemicals are toxic and are closing our kids' pores and not allowing their bodies to breathe properly. Long-term exposure to chemicals found in hygiene products, cosmetics, sunblock, fragrances, detergents, new carpets, vaccinations, and everyday household cleaners causes toxin overload. This stress causes the liver and adrenals to become diseased, but we do all of this because it's just easier and takes less time to grab a product without reading the labels.

Invest in your kids and know what is in the products they use every day—their brains and immune systems will thank you!! Children are now being born with elevated levels of chemicals in their umbilical cords. For example, two separate studies conducted in 2004 and 2008 by the Environmental Working Group (EWG) found 200+ environmental toxins in the umbilical cord blood from newborns. The issue isn't how many toxins are in your kid's system—sadly, they are present—but whether and/or how your kid's immune system reacts to them.

I also encourage you to learn more about the chemicals that are in vaccinations. Ty Bollinger presented some very valuable information about this in seven different episodes collectively called "The Truth about Vaccines." The information in his series is enough to write a book about. I am not going to go over all the details here, but I am asking you to take the time to educate yourself so you can make an informed decision for your child when it comes to the important matter of vaccines.

3. Spiritual Stress

When our kids are sick, where's our focus? Only on "My kid is sick!!"

Since you are taking the time to read this book, you must be ready to get your kid well. I am so proud of you right now!!

Making the time to read the Bible with your kids and listen to uplifting music can help empower your kid to live a purpose-filled life. Stress can come from confusion about what your kids believe. Your children may be confused about their purpose or why they are here—that alone can cause sickness. Going on mission trips can let your kids see how blessed they are.

4. Emotional Stress

Stress can result from a past experience like a divorce, the death of a close family member or friend, changing to a new school, or moving to a new house but not letting go of the old house and moving forward with life. It takes time to achieve emotional healing within.

Circular Stresses

The physical can affect the emotional in both of these ways:

- Glucose metabolism
- Brain function
- And there are more factors that can have cascading and circular effects on your kids:
- Food choices affect their emotional health,
- Their emotional health affects their relationships,
- Their relationships affect their physical and emotional health, and then…
- Their emotional and physical health can affect their food choices.
- But remember, there's no sense in being pessimistic—it wouldn't work, anyway!!
- When parents say "It can't be done," are they right? Or is it a matter of it can't be done by *them*?
- There is a basic flaw in the thinking of a pessimist, namely that "Nothing works!"
- If we take a pessimist's point of view, it would mean that there is no sense in being pessimistic, because it wouldn't work, anyway.
- Changing the way our kids think is key!
- The Bible says in Proverbs 23:7, "As a man thinks in his heart, so is he."

- Our kids will eventually become what they think—they can't think one thing and become something else.
- If we allow our kids to think negative, worried, fearful thoughts, then they will become negative, worried, fearful people. We cannot think defeat and expect victory.
- They can't think the worst and expect the best. They need to see themselves as being healthy kids who are thriving! Children learn and grow better when they put their energy toward what they can do rather than toward what they struggle to do.

We need to combat the idea of instant gratification.

- If it took your kid ten years to get in the state of health that they are in today, do you think it's only going to take ten days to get them out of it?

What's Important to You?

Everything you do is influenced by your values. In fact, values can cause a lot of your stress. Stress occurs when what you say you believe and what you actually do don't line up. For instance:

Most Americans would say the most important thing in life to them is:

- Family…
    - o BUT poll after poll after poll shows that the average father spends less than five minutes a day with his children. Still, these fathers would say "Family is number one."
    - o That's called incongruent values.

- Health…
    - o BUT when asked "Do you exercise?" and "Do you eat right?" and "Do you sleep right?" and "Do you take days off and rest?" the answer is always "No." But you probably still say "My kid's health is important to me."
    - o That's called incongruent values.

The 3 Rs for Combating Negative Thoughts

- Recognize where those thoughts come from.
    - o God does not put thoughts of anxiety and fear and worry into your kid's mind. Nice to know!!
- Reject the negative thought immediately.
    - o Don't even allow your kid to dwell on a negative thought for five seconds. The longer they think about it, the harder it's going to be to get rid of.
- Replace that thought instantly with the Truth—that is, with positive thoughts.

Remember, rejecting and recognizing are not enough, because if you don't replace that negative thought immediately, the same negativity will come back to your kid again and again and again.

Some may say to replace that negative thought with the Word of God. That principle still holds true.

Say this with me right now with your kid: "It's not my fault. I love, accept, and forgive myself."

I couldn't hear you. Say it out loud!!

"I love, accept, and forgive myself!!"

Now, say it again with me like you mean it: "I *love, accept*, and *forgive* myself."

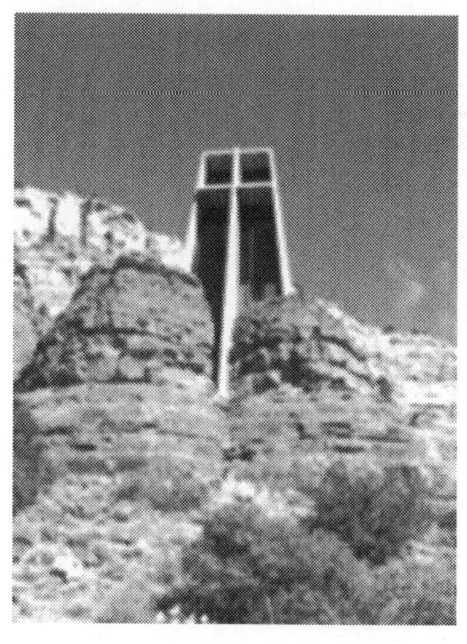

Man, that feels so good!! Take a *deep breath*!! Our children have to forgive themselves and other people in order to be healthy. I have a good friend who is an oncologist, and he once told me, "Dr. Corinne, the cause of cancer is unforgiveness." The first step in this is confession and receiving the forgiveness and restored fellowship that are the result of that confession (1 John 1:9). There is no doubt that God will bless our children and will glorify His name through it.

The word "forgive" comes from a Greek root word meaning "to set free or to let go." (I promise I won't start singing from Disney's *Frozen:* "Let it go, let it go!") To forgive, you must decide to give up any urges you have to be angry or resentful. Help your child disown those feelings and walk away from them. Set your child free and let go and let God be in control!

I know it's not easy, but that unforgiveness is a poison that is filling your child's body with sickness, so just love instead. Remember, forgiveness is not only something we do for other people—we do it for ourselves so we can get well and stay well.

Time Management

The statement I hear that bothers me the most is "Dr. Corinne, I don't have time." That's when I think, "Are you kidding me? It's all about priorities!" Remember, I have three kids and am a full-time doctor, speaker, and author. We all have to make time for what's important no matter how busy we are.

Here's a typical stressful scenario I see my clients causing again and again until I transform their thinking:

You are coming home after work and you're tired. Your kids need to eat, so you end up going to a drive-thru or ordering pizza because you don't feel like cooking. Not only does this type of food contribute to stress because of the poor-quality food, but now you feel guilty. ("My kids deserve healthy food!")

So then you give your kid some ice cream to feel better. They deserve it, right? But then your kid feels even worse because the dairy inflames their nasal passages and now they can't breathe as efficiently!! (And you know how I feel about breathing!)

Now the body isn't transporting oxygen to the cells as efficiently, so the brain isn't getting the oxygen it needs, and now your kid is depressed. Or the body has to pump the blood faster to get the oxygen to the cells, and that puts stress on your heart (this will affect blood pressure as well).

Now do you see why our kids are so stressed and sick?

Time-Saving Dinner Ideas (Yay!!)

Hippocrates said "Let food be thy medicine and medicine be thy food." When it comes to your child's health, your first and most crucial step is changing your kid's diet. This step is always the hardest because you must plan ahead of time—you can't just grab fast food and jump into doing the next thing on your list.

- Make crockpot meals: prepare the ingredients the night before in the ceramic part of the crock and then turn on the crockpot before you leave for work in the morning. A pressure cooker is also an awesome time-saving tool. My family loves cooking quinoa, rice, and sweet potatoes in it.

- Cook extra chicken to make a chicken salad later or to use in soups and casseroles for lunch or dinner the next day.
- Most grocery stores now carry very good organic salad mixes. I always have a bag on hand for an easy side salad at dinnertime or as a quick lunch salad. (Since my lovely husband works at Costco, we get all of our organic lettuce there.)
- "Baking" sweet potatoes in a crockpot or pressure cooker is easy—they turn out fantastic!
    - Place clean potatoes in crock pot and cook on HIGH for about 3 hours…
    - Or place about a cup of water in the bottom of a pressure cooker, put the potato in a steamer basket and set it inside the cooker, bring to pressure, and cook for 12-15 minutes. (Timing may vary for different cookers and different amounts of potatoes.) Remember, it's up to you as parents to change your own thinking, too. I know you love your family and want what's best for them. Your heart's desire is to improve your child's immune system so they can achieve their best brain potential. You can do this!!
- When you're at home, you've got to eat the best you can, because sometimes you don't have control over what you eat (as in when you are eating away from home).
- Also, learn how to make better choices when you eat out. Our favorite fast-food restaurant is Chipotle; our kids love it there. We get the burrito bowl with no cheese or sour cream—we add guacamole instead.

Use this type of common sense about restaurant meals, but be open-minded and disciplined enough to know when things are getting out of hand, like when you need to eat at home more often.

Foods to Avoid: Bad Fats

We need good dietary fats for our kids' brains and development. Fats from fish, nuts, seeds, olive oil, and coconut oil are good for you (unless your kid is allergic to any of these). Fats to limit or avoid entirely are saturated fats (except for coconut and palm oils) and trans fats. Cheeses, ice cream, dairy products, meats, and shortening contain substantial amounts of saturated fats, while baked goods are generally loaded with trans fats. However, high-quality coconut oil—although rich in saturated fat—no longer carries the stigma it once did. It has many health benefits and should be used for high-temperature frying.

Facts about hydrogenated or "trans" fats:

- Trans fats do not exist in nature.
- Trans fats are the hardest fat for our bodies to correctly break down.
- Trans fats lead to digestive problems.
- Trans fats have the capacity to do more harm than saturated fats do.

What contains hydrogenated or trans fats?

- Margarines, most prepackaged foods and dressings, and products containing Olestra.
- Almost every processed food in the supermarket contains trans fats: soups, chips, crackers, cookies, pastries, mixes of all kinds, even including some pasta and rice mixes.
- Frozen foods like pizzas and pot pies and even some cereals are made with trans fats.
- Deep-fried foods such as donuts, French fries, breaded chicken and fish, etc. are often fried in trans fats.

To avoid bad fats, look for the words "hydrogenated," "partially hydrogenated," "trans fatty acids," or "trans fats", and "interestified" on ingredient labels. Put those products back on the shelf!

Foods to Avoid: Sugar

I know—sugar is in everything. But avoid all sugars and sweeteners! When you have a sick kid, you become a crazy person because you're looking at every food label before you hand that food to your kid to eat. I mean, really, there is so much artificial crap in our food. No wonder our kids are sick and their brains are hypersensitive! We must be on guard at all times, because people love handing out candy and sodas to our kids. I don't understand why every holiday has to be surrounded by sugar. Come on, people! When are we going to realize that fake, sugar-filled food is making us sick??

More importantly, sugar inflames everything, including our kids' brains. We don't have desserts in my family's house, or if we do, it's usually organic frozen fruit or a piece of dark chocolate with coconut chips.

Foods to Avoid: Caffeine

Remember, caffeine includes energy drinks! Caffeine is a drug that causes anxiety, fatigue, and depression, all of which leads to more stress for your child. When people suffer from anxiety, the more caffeine they consume, the more anxious and depressed they feel.

Double-blind studies have shown that people with anxiety often experience worse symptoms of anxiety after ingesting caffeine. In addition, suddenly stopping regular caffeine ingestion may temporarily worsen anxiety.

Foods to Avoid: Dairy and Gluten

Dairy and gluten cause weight gain and affect sinus and breathing issues. Both can make children chronically sick, especially kids with brain dysfunction. Remember: just breathe!!

Does Today's Milk Do Our Body Good?

As a kid, we loved making milkshakes and having milk mustaches like the celebrities did. Remember those ads telling us to drink milk? ("Milk—it makes a body strong!") Little did my parents know that milk was causing my body not to heal! The dairy industry sure did an excellent job of marketing milk to us as a reliable source of calcium and a way to make our bodies strong.

But milk isn't what those ads made it out to be. Modern feeding methods for cows substitute high-protein, soy-based feeds for fresh green grass; in addition, modern breeding methods produce cows with abnormally large pituitary glands. Why is that done? So that the cows can produce three times more milk than the old-fashioned cow used to be able to. These cows also need regular doses of antibiotics to keep them well.

Other issues with today's milk:

- The pasteurization process destroys all valuable enzymes (without these, milk is very difficult to digest):
  - Lactase for the assimilation of lactose.
  - Galactase for the assimilation of galactose.
  - Phosphatase for the assimilation of calcium.
  - The human pancreas is not always able to produce these enzymes, and overstressing the pancreas can lead to diabetes and other diseases.

- Skim milk is sold as a health food; however, butterfat is in milk for a reason.
  - o Without butterfat, the body cannot absorb and utilize the vitamins and minerals in the water fraction of the milk.
  - o Synthetic vitamin D—which known to be toxic to the liver—is added to conventional skim milk to replace the natural vitamin D complex found in butterfat.
  - o Butterfat also contains properties which have strong anti-carcinogenic properties.
- Pus + hormones = milk.
  - o The USDA does not allow milk containing 750 million or more pus cells per liter to be shipped across state borders. However, author Jim Dickrell reports that the level of pus cells has been rising ever since farmers began using Monsanto's genetically engineered bovine growth hormone.
- Allergies
  - o "Formula-fed babies, at the age of three months, were secreting low levels of serum antibodies to bovine proteins contained in their formula (5)."
  - o "Most formula-fed infants developed symptoms of *allergic* rejection to cow milk proteins before one month of age. About 50-70% experienced rashes or other skin symptoms, 50-60% gastrointestinal symptoms, and 20-30% respiratory symptoms. The recommended therapy is to avoid cow's milk (6)."
- Calcium deficiency
  - o Despite the country's large consumption of dairy products, one out of every two American women over 50 will have an osteoporosis-related fracture in her lifetime.
  - o Most the world's population takes in less than half the calcium we are told we need, yet they have strong bones

and healthy teeth while our kids' teeth are full of cavities. I had a dad tell me yesterday that his son's dentist told him he has many dental issues today due to overexposure of antibiotics he was on for his ear infections.

- o Is it possible to obtain all your calcium from dark green vegetables? Yes!!! The darker, the better!!

Sources of calcium

- 1 ounce of cheese: 207 mg
- 8 ounces of milk: 300 mg

Now look at these alternatives and the amount of calcium that is in them!

- 1 cup cooked collard greens: 266 mg
- 1 cup rice milk (plain, calcium-fortified): 200-300 mg
- 1 cup cooked turnip greens: 197 mg
- 1 cup cooked black-eyed peas: 211 mg
- 1 cup cooked kale: 94 mg
- 2 tablespoons sesame seeds: 176 mg
- 1 cup cooked okra: 176 mg
- 1 cup boiled bok choy: 186 mg
- 1 tablespoon blackstrap molasses: 137 mg
- 5 medium dried figs: 135 mg
- 1/4 cup almonds: 97 mg
- 1 cup cooked broccoli: 100 mg
- 1/2 cup cooked amaranth: 74 mg
- 1/2 cup dried apricots: 43 mg
- 1/2 cup cooked quinoa: 30 mg
- FYI: maple syrup has twice as much calcium as milk! (but don't let your child drink 3 glasses per day!)

- By far the best source of calcium is small fish, because you can eat the bones: herring, sardines, anchovies, etc. Bonus: those fish are also rich in omega-3 fats and don't contain sugar.

Dairy Substitutions

Milk

- o 1 cup = 1 cup of rice milk, almond milk, coconut milk

Buttermilk

- o 1 cup = 1 cup minus 1 tablespoon of rice milk, almond milk, flax milk, hemp milk, or coconut milk plus 1 tablespoon of lemon juice (let set for a few minutes to thicken before using)

Butter

- o 1 tablespoon = 1 tablespoon sunflower or palm oil (baking is an exception due to water %)

Heavy cream

- o 1 tablespoon = 1 tablespoon coconut cream

Replacing Bad Food Habits with Exercise

Replace the stimulatory caffeine and sugar with good ol' exercise!

Benefits of exercise that you may not know:

- Greater mental clarity.
- Detox!

- Improves insulin receptor sensitivity, meaning that your insulin resistance will decrease and you'll have lower insulin levels, which makes it much easier to burn fat.
- www.physicalbreathing.com
    - o Visit my site, and I will send you an exercise plan you can do with your child for free. Let's get physical, physical, physical! Let me hear your body talk!! Go grab some bands and do some back exercises with your child that you'll find in my book *Learning How to Breathe.*

Change your attitude about exercise. Exercise isn't just good for weight loss—it also boosts your child's brain health and mental clarity (and yours, too!). I just love jumping on the trampoline with my kids, or taking a walk, riding bikes, or playing tennis.

Foods to Include: Fats

A lot of times, people ask me "What are good fats?" I love to tell them about omega fats!

- Omega-3 fats are good fats. They can be found in raw nuts and seeds as well as in beans, fish oil, and avocado as well as unrefined flax, hemp, and walnut oils.
- Omega-6 fats are also good fats and are in certain vegetable oils such as safflower, sunflower, olive, grapeseed, and sesame.

What role do fats play in health?

- Fats keep cell membranes fluid and flexible, which in turn boosts the white blood cells that repel invaders out of the body.

- Fats also build your child's immune system and brain.
- Fats promote normal growth for your child, especially of blood vessels and nerves (i.e., helps their bodies repair themselves).
- Fats keep the skin and other tissues healthy and smooth.
- Our children can't live fat-free lives: they need significant amounts of essential fatty acids to function properly and to enhance their brain function and immunity.

Also, attention, ladies who are pregnant or nursing! Take EPA/DHA-rich fish oil (3000 mg) and GLA-rich flax oil (240 mg) every night before you go to bed!

Nutty Statistics

- All nuts contain arginine, an amino acid that helps keep arteries clear. Nuts also contain magnesium and potassium, which are associated with lowered blood pressure.
- Compared to other nuts, almonds top the list for calcium, fiber, and Vitamin E content.
- Brazil nuts from Brazil not grown in China have more calcium than milk and are high in selenium (an antioxidant). Also, it's easy to overdo it on the high amounts of selenium found in Brazil nuts from Brazil. Caution: Don't eat too many—a selenium overdose makes you feel pretty sick.
- Pistachios have more fiber than broccoli. Maybe your child would like pistachios better!
- Pumpkin seeds are a reliable source of zinc, which helps promote fertility and cellular reproduction, supports vision and immunity, and protects against free radicals.

- Raw, unsalted nuts are a better option than roasted, unsalted nuts.
- Watch out for hydrogenated fats used in the roasting process!

Hydrogenated Fat Substitutions

- Earth Balance spread (butter substitute)
- Extra-virgin olive oil (must be extra-virgin)
- Spectrum brand shortening
- Sunflower oil
- Safflower oil
- Avocado oil
- Grapeseed oil
- Note: Canola oil is not a good-quality oil. It is cheap, but it goes rancid quickly (even at very low temperatures) and is genetically modified.
- Note: sunflower, safflower, and grapeseed oils are also very heavily processed, high in omega-6s rather than 3s, and are very inflammatory so use olive oil and avocado oils more often.

Foods to Include: Honey

I love our Dancing Bees honey—it's organic and pure (you can buy it at www.dr.corinneweaver.com).

- Honey keeps well and never spoils.
- Dieters, take notice!
  - o Dextrose is assimilated very quickly, giving that "instant" boost of energy the body needs.

- o Levulose is absorbed much more slowly and maintains blood sugar levels for some time.
- o Honey's double-action combination of sugars quickly satisfies a craving for sweets and tends to maintain a sense of satisfaction for a while.

- Honey has anti-bacterial properties.

Foods to Include: Nutritional Yeast

- This is not the same as the yeast in bread and will not contribute to yeast infections.
- It's high in B-complex vitamins.
- Sprinkle in casseroles and soups for a "cheesy" or savory flavor.

The Many Roles of Food

Food plays a role in many aspects of your child's life, from celebration to sorrow. The last thing you want is a long-term rigid list of rules about what to eat. Good nutrition is more than just rules! No matter the basis of your personal food decisions, finding balance and peace with food is key to a lifetime of good health and well-being.

Information-based decisions are the most important aspects of a healthy diet, which is a diet that involves making choices that allow for flexibility rather than just following rigid dietary rules. In fact, strict dietary rules often lead to failure in the long run…and it's the long run that you must always be thinking about when it comes to your diet.

Here is a useful thought that you can build upon based on your own experience and self-education: to have health like no one else, you must live like no one else.

Consider the "big picture" and evaluate success over time from many perspectives.

- Always return to your core. If you have a cheat, don't let that become the new norm! Don't allow compromises to add up in your fridge or pantry, either—always keep your head in the game.
- Open your mind to healthy foods such as fruits, vegetables, lean meats, and healthy fats. Set small, achievable goals and make changes that you can live with for the long run. Consider what your family needs, and if your plan doesn't work, don't give up—adjust!
- Buying organic is one way to help you stay away from more chemicals, which is a stressor to our bodies.

Organic Produce

- Is grown without synthetic fertilizers or irradiation
- Is not genetically engineered or modified
- Is grown without chemical pesticides
- Is grown in high-quality soil
- Is grown using natural pest and weed control (better for the environment and for us!)
- Contains more vitamins, antioxidants, and phytonutrients

Grass-Fed/Pastured Meat and Dairy Animals

- Must be raised under specific animal welfare guidelines
- Cannot be given antibiotics or growth hormones, but when the animals are sick, they are given antibiotics and removed from the general population to recover.
- Must be provided with access to the outdoors but sadly this can be a tiny trapdoor leading to an asphalt parking lot.
- Must be fed with 100% organic feed but the feed could still be corn and soy
- Cannot be fed animal byproducts or genetically modified (GMO) crops
- Must be fed/produced on land that has been free from the use of toxic and persistent chemical pesticides and fertilizers for a minimum of three years
- Are a humane way to raise animals
- Are better for the environment
- Note: Bear in mind that that there is NO official third-party certification for grass-fed/pastured products the way there is for organic. Very important to know this.

Free-Range/Pastured Hens

- Many free-range operations do not bother to become certified organic
- Must be fed organic feed but again can be corn and soy
- May not receive any antibiotics but when the animals are sick, they are given antibiotics and removed from the general population to recover.

- Must be allowed access to the outdoors and raised in a cage-free environment but sadly this can be a tiny trapdoor leading to an asphalt parking lot.
- Are a humane way to raise animals
- Note: Bear in mind that that there is NO official third-party certification for grass-fed/pastured products the way there is for organic. Very important to know this.

Understanding Organic Food Labels, Benefits, and Claims

Before I get into all the logistics of organic food just know there are small local farmers that often use organic methods but sometimes cannot afford to become certified organic. Visit a farmer's market and talk with the farmers around you. Find out how they produce the fruits and vegetables they sell. You can even ask for a farm tour, which I have done before with my kids. They loved seeing the gardens and petting the animals, **just know the farmers are very busy and plan a visit ahead of time.**

Organic Farms

- Farms must undergo USDA inspection and certification to bear the organic seal
- Handlers and processors who work with the food before it reaches the market must be organic-certified as well
- Meat marketed as "organic" must be 100% organic
- Multi-ingredient products marketed with the USDA organic seal must contain 95% or more certified organic content

Organic food has become very popular, but navigating the maze of organic food labels, benefits, and claims can be confusing. Is organic food healthier? Is it more nutritious? What do all the labels mean? Why is it so expensive? This guide can help you make better choices about which organic foods are healthier for your family and better for the environment and how you can afford to incorporate more organic food into your family's diet.

Making a commitment to healthy eating is a great start towards a healthier life, in part because healthy foods help you breathe better. Beyond eating more fruits, vegetables, whole and gluten-free grains, and good fats, however, there are the questions of food safety, nutrition, and sustainability. How foods are grown or raised can impact both your health and the environment. This brings up more questions: what is the difference between organic foods and conventionally grown foods? Is organic always best? What about locally grown foods?

What Are Genetically Modified Organisms (GMOs)?

Genetically modified organisms (GMOs) are plants or animals whose DNA has been altered. These products have undergone only short-term testing to determine their effects on humans and the environment. In most countries, organic products do not contain GMOs.

The Benefits of Organic Food

Organic foods provide a variety of benefits. Some studies show that organic foods have more beneficial nutrients (such as antioxidants) than their conventionally grown counterparts do. In addition, people with allergies to foods, chemicals, or preservatives often find their symptoms lessen or go away when they eat only organic foods.

Organic produce contains fewer pesticides, fungicides, herbicides, and insecticides. These chemicals are widely used in conventional agriculture, and residues remain on (and in) the food we eat.

Here's a great tip: conventional produce has 4-digit codes. GMO versions of that same produce have 5 digits starting with an 8. Organic versions have 5-digit codes starting with a 9. For example: a conventional Braeburn is 4101; a GMO Braeburn (which I don't think exists—I'm just using this as an example) would be 84101; an organic Braeburn would be 94101.

Why Do Pesticides Matter?

Children and fetuses are most vulnerable to pesticide exposure due to their less-developed immune systems and because their bodies and brains are still developing. Exposure at an early age can cause developmental delays, behavioral disorders, respiratory issues, and motor dysfunction.

Pregnant women are more vulnerable due to the added stress pesticides put on their already taxed organs. Plus, pesticides can be passed from mother to child in the womb as well as through breast milk. Some exposures can cause delayed effects on the nervous system years after the initial exposure.

Most of us have an **accumulated build-up** of pesticide exposure in our bodies due to numerous years of exposure. This chemical "body burden," as it is medically known, can lead to health issues such as headaches, birth defects, and an added strain on weakened immune systems.

Organic food is often fresher. Fresh food tastes better. Organic food is usually fresher because it doesn't contain preservatives that would make it last longer. Organic produce is often—but not always, so watch where it is from—produced on smaller farms near where it is sold.

Organic farming is better for the environment. Organic farming practices reduce pollution (air, water, soil), conserve water, reduce soil erosion, increase soil fertility, and use less energy. In addition, organic farming is better for birds and small animals, as chemical pesticides can make it harder for these creatures to reproduce; pesticides can even kill them. Farming without pesticides is also better for the farmworkers who harvest our food.

Organically raised animals are not given routine antibiotics or growth hormones, nor are they fed animal byproducts. The use of routine antibiotics in conventional meat production helps create antibiotic-resistant strains of bacteria. This means that when someone gets sick from these strains, they will be less responsive to antibiotic treatment.

Not feeding animal byproducts to other animals reduces the risk of mad cow disease (BSE). In addition, organically raised animals are given more space to move around and access to the outdoors, both of which help to keep the animals healthy. The more crowded the conditions, the more likely an animal is to get sick. Technically, the "access to the outdoors" requirement can be a tiny hatch door that leads to an asphalt parking lot. It's unfortunately one of those loosey-goosey requirements that can be loop holed. Pastured/grass-fed is a far better option assuming that you could verify that the farm is indeed pastured/grass-fed. Such farms may or may not take on the effort and cost of becoming certified organic.

Organic Farming and Locally Grown Produce

Organic farming refers to the agricultural production systems that are used to produce food and fiber. Organic farmers don't use synthetic pesticides or fertilizers—instead, they rely on biological diversity in the field to naturally reduce habitat for pest organisms. Organic farmers also purposefully maintain and replenish the fertility of the soil. All kinds of agricultural products are produced organically, including produce, grains, meat, dairy, eggs, fibers such as cotton, flowers, and processed food products.

Essential Characteristics of Organic Systems

- Design and implementation of an "organic system plan" that describes the practices used in producing crops and livestock products.
- Detailed record-keeping systems that track all products from the field to the point of sale.
- Maintenance of buffer zones to prevent inadvertent contamination by synthetic farm chemicals from adjacent conventional fields.

Organic vs. Non-Organic Produce	
Organic Produce:	Conventionally Grown Produce:
No pesticides	Pesticides used
Grown with natural fertilizers (manure, compost)	Grown with synthetic or chemical fertilizers
Weeds are controlled naturally (crop rotation, hand-weeding, mulching, and tilling)	Weeds are controlled with chemical herbicides
Insects are controlled using natural methods (birds, good insects, traps)	Insecticides are used to manage pests and disease

Locally Grown Fruits and Veggies

What is "local" food? Unlike organic standards, there is no specific definition. Generally, local food means food that was grown close to home. This could be in your own garden, your local community, your state, your region, or your country. During substantial portions of the year, it is usually possible to find food grown very close to home at places like a farmer's market. I enjoy getting to know my local farmers and supporting the ones who do their best to provide the best-quality organic food.

There are great financial benefits to buying locally. Money stays within the community, for example, and strengthens the local economy. More money goes directly to the farmer instead of to marketers and distributors.

Also, when you buy local, you are helping keep our air clean. In the US, for example, the average meal travels over 1,500 miles from the farm to the dinner plate. This long journey uses a lot of fossil fuels and emits carbon dioxide into the air, causing more breathing issues. In addition, some produce must be picked while still unripe and then gassed to "ripen" it after transport. Some produce is highly processed in factories using preservatives, irradiation, and other means to keep it stable for transport and sale.

Local food is the freshest food you can purchase. Fruits and vegetables are harvested when they are ripe and full of flavor—very yummy!

If you want garden-fresh produce but don't have a green thumb or time to invest in having your own garden, consider a CSA agreement (Community Supported Agriculture). The "bang for your buck" is incredible, and you get to try new veggies and fruits every time your order comes in!

Fruits and vegetables where the organic label matters most	
According to the Environmental Working Group, a nonprofit organization that analyzes the results of government pesticide testing in the US, the following 12 commercially grown fruits and vegetables ("The Dirty Dozen") have the highest pesticide levels on average. Because of their high pesticide levels, it is best to buy these organic. The list does change every year so go to www.ewg.org to find the updated changes. Here is 2017.	
Apples	Pears
Sweet Bell peppers	Peaches
Spinach	Nectarines
Celery	Tomatoes
Cherries	Potatoes
Grapes	Strawberries

Non-organic fruits and vegetables with low pesticide levels	
These conventionally grown 15 fruits and vegetables ("The Clean Fifteen") were found to have the lowest levels of pesticides—most of them have a thicker skin or peel, which naturally protects them better from pests and means their production does not require the use of as many pesticides. The list does change every year so go to www.ewg.org to find the updated changes. Here is 2017.	
Asparagus	Onions
Avocados	Papayas
Honeydew Melon	Pineapples
Cabbage	Peas (sweet)
Corn (sweet)	Cantaloupe
Eggplant	Cauliflower
Kiwi	Grapefruit
Mangoes	

Does Washing and Peeling Get Rid of Pesticides?

Rinsing reduces—but does not eliminate!—pesticides. Peeling sometimes helps, but valuable nutrients often go down the drain with the skin. The best approach is to eat a varied diet, wash all produce, and buy organic whenever possible.

You can make your own veggie/fruit wash with lemon essential oil. I fill a clean big pot with water, add 5 drops of lemon essential oil and soak them for 20-30 minutes. You can also use 1/2 cup of white vinegar and not lemon oil. Sometimes I combine the two. The lemon oil removes the wax and toxins and keeps the produce fresh.

Organic Meat and Dairy

Organic meat, dairy products, and eggs are produced from animals that are fed organic feed (which may be corn and soy) and allowed access to the outdoors, even though it is very limited. They must be kept in living conditions that accommodate the natural behavior of the animals, such as ruminants having access to pasture. Organic livestock and poultry may not be given antibiotics, hormones, or medications in the absence of illness; however, they may be vaccinated against disease. Parasiticide (a substance or agent used to destroy parasites) use is strictly regulated. Livestock diseases and parasites are controlled primarily through preventative measures such as rotational grazing, balanced diets, sanitary housing, and stress reduction.

Organic vs. Conventional Meat and Dairy	
Regulations governing meat and dairy farming vary from country to country. In the US, these meat and dairy products from conventionally raised animals were found to have the lowest levels of pesticides. Again, getting local farmers meat is the best. Do your homework in your local area to see what farmers are doing their best to raise animals organically.	
Organic meat and dairy: No antibiotics, hormones, or pesticides are given to the animals Livestock are given all organic feed Disease is prevented with natural methods such as clean housing, rotational grazing, and a healthy diet Livestock must have access to the outdoors	Conventionally raised meat and dairy: Typically given antibiotics, hormones and feed containing ingredients grown with pesticides Livestock are given growth hormones for faster growth Antibiotics and medications are used to prevent livestock disease Livestock may or may not have access to the outdoors

Buying Tips for Organic Foods

Buy in season! Fruits and vegetables are cheapest and freshest when they are in season. You can also find out when produce is delivered to your market. That way, you know you're buying the freshest food possible.

Shop around! Compare the price of organic items at the grocery store, the produce market, the farmer's market, and any other venue (even in the freezer aisle!). Purchase the most economical ones. If local foods are not available, we shop at Costco and Trader Joe's. These two stores are the most reasonable in price when you are buying organic in bulk. Having three kids means buying food all the time, so I am so thankful my husband works at Costco, because I am always telling him to bring this and that home.

But remember: organic doesn't always equal healthy! Junk food can just as easily be made using organic ingredients. Making junk food sound healthy is a common marketing ploy in the food industry, but organic baked goods, desserts, and snacks are usually still very high in sugar, salt, fat, and/or calories.

Make the Switch to Better Food

- Slowly eliminate sugar and caffeine.
- Replace these stimulants with exercise.
    - Exercise with your child!
- Start slow and develop new habits one at a time.
    - Keep focused on your child's long-term development.
- Attend our Wellness Kid webinars and classes to build fellowship with like-minded individuals, get on our email list for announcements, and become a Wellness member for added support.

Don't Guess About Your Child's Health!

- It's clear we cannot get all the nutrients we need from food for our kids' optimal body functioning and wellness.
- The only way to know what your children need and how much they need is to have them properly tested for Nutritional deficiencies.
- We test! This is why I see success when I treat many childhood health disorders.

In the next chapter, I will discuss the "T" in my S-T-R-E-S-S system, which stands for "testing and therapies."

Have a question for me? Send me your health concerns and connect with me. I want to know what you think! You can reach me at:

www.drcorinneweaver.com/index.php/apply-now/

where you can apply to be a client

Action Item:

What do you see in your child's future?

1) ____

____

____

____

____

____

____

____

____

____

____

Chapter 4

T-ESTING AND THERAPIES

The second letter of my S-T-R-E-S-S system is "T" for "*T-esting and therapies*." What tests should I do for my kid and why? Here are the tests I have found to be very helpful: thermography, food allergy test, hair and blood test, stool test, neurological exam, upper-cervical-specific X-rays, adrenal/hormone test, and EEG brain map. Which therapies work? Upper cervical care, BEMER vascular, neuromuscular massage, music, physical breathing, aromatherapy, exercise, laughter, prayer, nutritional support, and neurofeedback.

Thermography

The first step is to identify the inflammation in your child's body so that we can start removing what is causing their body to be inflamed. We can use thermographic analysis to determine if your child has any inflammation in their nerves, lungs, sinuses, or gut.

As a doctor, I want to have a diagnostic tool to assist me in finding inflammation and knowing when and when not to correct the spine. Thermography is the best tool to show the physiology of the body's inflamed areas. Full-body thermographic scans for men, women, and children are valuable tools for preventative health monitoring that assists with the early detection and analysis of abnormal vascular activity, inflammation, and pain throughout the body.

Thermography is a painless, noninvasive screening test that converts infrared radiation emitted from the skin surface into electrical impulses, which are visualized in color on a computer monitor. This visual image is a graphic map of body temperature; it is referred to as a thermogram.

Thermograms show a spectrum of colors and can indicate an increase or decrease in the amount of infrared radiation being emitted from the body's surface. Since a normal body has a high degree of thermal symmetry, any subtle abnormal temperature asymmetry (which typically accompanies inflammation, infection, injury, or disease) can easily be identified.

The advantage of using this method of early detection is that it establishes a baseline for changes in your health, baseline that can help prevent future health issues. There is no exposure to radiation and no physical contact with the camera. It is completely nonionizing, safe, and can be repeated as often as required without exposing the patient to risk.

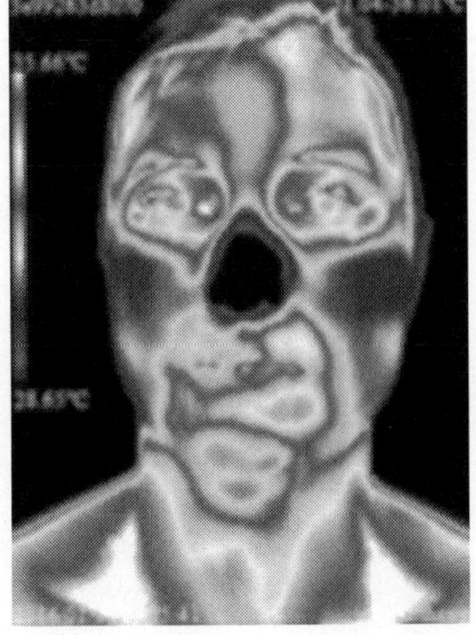

Here is a face shot of me with thermography. Since the book is in black and white, you will have to go to my website to see it in color. Thermography not only shows inflammation in the nerve patterns, lungs, sinuses, and gut, we also use it for breast health awareness. (With every thermography we do in our office, we give away Olivia Newton-John's breast self-exam kit called the Liv Kit. The Liv Kit is a tool you can place over your breast to help you easily detect breast lumps. Every woman should be doing breast self-exams: you know your body the best, and the more familiar you get with your body, the more you will know when there's a problem or when something doesn't feel right.)

Techniques to Ease Inflammation

At our office, we give you a plan of action for your child after your thermography results come back in. Here is a sample of some advice we give to our patients.

If your child's muscles are inflamed in their jaw and neck, we recommend applying lavender oil to their jaw joint and doing some neck stretches along with receiving upper cervical care.

If their diaphragm muscle is very tight, we recommend lying with a half foam roll or a towel rolled up under their lower back and doing deep breathing exercises. We encourage inhaling through the nose for a count of 4-8 and then exhaling through the nose for a count of 4-8 while placing one hand on chest and one hand on abdomen to encourage diaphragm breathing. (The hand on the chest should remain still while the hand on the abdomen should rise and fall with each breath.) If you have them close their eyes while doing this, their muscles will be able to better relax. The goal is 6-10 breaths per minute for 10 minutes a day.

Another relaxing technique for your child is soaking in an Epsom salt bath one to two times a week. I recommend adding ¼ cup of Epsom salt to the bath along with 2 drops of lavender essential oil.

Thyroid Issues

If the thyroid is showing cold or very hot patterns, we recommend having some bloodwork done to get a full thyroid evaluation for your child.

Sinus Congestion

If the thermography shows sinus congestion, we recommend applying melaleuca, peppermint, and eucalyptus essential oils behind both ears or feet (depending on your child's age) and doing the massage technique below. Always make sure you dilute. You can dilute pure essential oils with carrier oil in a ratio of 1 part essential oil to 2 parts carrier oil and put it in a handy roller bottle.

Massaging your child's sinuses and tissues can help relieve pressure and drain any mucus-filled sinus cavities. Don't get the oils in your child's eyes when doing this massage! Have them keep their eyes closed and use your thumbs to apply the right amount of pressure (i.e., pressure that doesn't cause intense pain) starting at the frontal sinuses on their forehead. Rub in a circular motion 10-15 times, then rub between the eyes and massage in a circular motion around the eyes for 1-2 minutes. Next, apply pressure under the cheekbones starting at the nose and going towards the ears. Apply firm and constant pressure for 1-2 minutes. (You can see a video of how to do this on my YouTube channel.) Lastly, steep some peppermint or eucalyptus tea, place a large kitchen towel over your child's head, and have them breathe in the tea steam for 5-10 minutes while staying about 15 inches away from the pot. Do these routines every hour if needed to help relieve the congestion. These techniques helped me when I got sinus infections.

Sometimes a child may need a nasal-specific technique performed (especially children like me who took a fall to the face). Accidents and injuries to the face and head can cause the bones of the skull to shift and thereby increase the pressure in our skull, affecting our brain and nervous system. My brother's nose was broken when he was hit by a baseball bat as a kid, and consequently he was not breathing at all through his nose. I learned the following procedure to help him breathe, then had it performed on myself.

There is a way to adjust the bones of the skull, specifically the sphenoid bone. The procedure is done by inserting small balloons into each of your child's six nasal passages and gently inflating them so the passageways can open. This procedure is not the most pleasant, but it can be life-changing for children who can't breathe through their nose. My brother and other patients who have struggled to breathe through their noses have thanked me for learning this technique. Most children notice immediate improvement in their ability to breathe! Now I, too, can fully breathe through my nose.

Liver and Gut Issues

If your child's liver and gut are very inflamed, we recommend starting with colloidal bentonite and fiber with psyllium seed/husk. On the first night, have your child take 1/4 cup of the liquid bentonite and swish it in their mouth, then swallow. Continue with 2 tablespoons each morning and night (leave liquid in mouth for 1-3 minutes like you would a mouthwash, then swallow). Bentonite clay is a natural detoxifier and helps carries heavy metals out of our body, thereby improving immunity and reducing inflammation. It also kills bacteria and viruses. The clay comes from ash taken from volcanoes and contains beneficial trace minerals that we need. We also recommend applying bentonite clay mixed with water to a cotton ball and putting it on inflamed gum sites for 15 minutes a day.

After you have completed 30 days of using the colloidal bentonite, we recommend coconut oil pulling in the morning. I recommend using 1-3 teaspoons of coconut oil and swishing it in the mouth for 3-5 minutes. Coconut has antibacterial properties and helps to clean the bad bacteria from the mouth.

I also recommend a liver and gall bladder cleanse. A liver cleanse helps your child balance hormones and removes toxins from their body, which decreases congestion of lymph in the chest/breasts. Performing a quarterly detox is recommended to assist the body in clearing toxins and preventing the body from storing toxins.

Detoxing

The detoxes I recommend quarterly are called Clear Change by Metagenics and Core Restore by Orthomolecular. My patients are glad I use these easier cleanses now, because the one my Uncle John recommended was a 7-10 day fast with just fiber and herbs. That was my very first detox, and I did it when my oldest child, Noah, was only one year old. It was very hard.

More information can be found on cweaver.metagenics.com or www.drcorinneweaver.com.

Lymph Congestion

For lymph congestion, I recommend dry brushing. Dry brushing helps stimulate your child's lymph system and encourages removal of toxins. To do this, you need a medium-soft skin brush. Start at the feet and brush upward towards the heart. Use firm—but not too hard—and small strokes in a circular motion. Dedicate 3-5 minutes to brushing the whole body. The kids and I do it in the morning before we shower and have noticed increased energy because the brushing also helps stimulate blood flow. A rush of energy is always a good thing in the morning! Do not forget to apply a good natural lotion afterwards. Your child's skin will thank you!

Rebounding is also fun to do for lymph congestion, although it does require at least a small rebounder trampoline. I have a big trampoline in the backyard, so when I am jumping around and having fun with the kids, I am also helping my lymph system—extra bonus points! (My girls keep me accountable for doing this, because it is a special time with them to jump and share girl talk.) I recommend rebounding for 15 minutes a day. A modified version of this involves sitting and bouncing on an exercise ball for 15 minutes a day. Both methods are fun and effective.

Another way to stimulate your child's lymph system is to lightly beat on the chest area like Tarzan. (The thymus gland is in the center of the chest and is part of the immune system.) After your children do their dry brushing, they can beat on their chest like Tarzan in the shower! I know you're probably thinking I am silly, but there is a lot of truth in my words. If you really want to go crazy, rub diluted peppermint oil onto their chest. That will wake them up, get them going for the day, and help them to stay focused.

Boosting Blood Flow

Another great tool I use to boost blood flow is the BEMER mat. This benefits the cardiac system, the body's regenerative abilities, and even mental acuity. It is a mat you lay on that uses a Pulsed Electro Magnetic Field (PEMF) to increase blood flow. Today, the only similarity between PEMF and BEMER devices is the electro-magnetic field. However, the BEMER doesn't use PEMF as an active agent, but as a carrier for its unique physical signal configuration. The BEMER Group owns five global patents and has received numerous scientific awards for its research. The BEMER mat enhances general blood flow, the body's nutrient and oxygen supply, and waste disposal. It also helps with stress reduction and relaxation. It is a wonderful tool to use for babies and children, and it only takes 8 minutes a day. It increases their cellular level of healing and helps the body regenerate after an injury. It is also used by NASA astronauts to improve bone and muscle atrophy during space missions. That is so cool!!

For more information, you can go to:

http://drweaver.bemergroup.com/en-US.

Digestion Distress

For digestion distress, I recommend taking 1-2 tablespoons of apple cider vinegar before meals. If apple cider vinegar is new to your child, start with 1 teaspoon and mix with small amount of water and honey if desired. I also recommend taking digestive enzymes, increasing your fiber (1 teaspoon of psyllium seed/husk per day), and taking probiotics. For psyllium, I love using Ready! Set! Go! from Orthomolecular products. The American Heart Association recommends that children consume between 19 and 31 grams of fiber per day depending on their age. A lack of fiber intake can lead to constipation, gas, and bloating. The formula Ready! Set! Go! has psyllium in it, along with all-natural fruit and plant extracts to help relieve constipation and soothe an achy stomach. Also, it tastes great!!

Sometimes on the thermography scan, inflammation shows up where the pyloric valve is. I have found pyloric valve exercises to be very helpful for kids. The pyloric valve is between the stomach and the small intestine and is located 2 inches up from the belly button. It plays a significant role in digestion because it controls the flow of food. If the valve is not working properly, we have all kinds of digestive symptoms (one of them being acid reflux). When our kids feel threatened, their digestive systems shut down or greatly slow down, slowing this valve. Stress can cause all kinds of problems, including digestive issues. To get this valve working properly again, you can do a release exercise.

When starting the release, start slowly, breathe deeply, and do the release several hours after eating in evening. For more details, see the pyloric valve release instructional video on my YouTube channel.

Some of my goals for sick kids as they follow the above recommendations are these:

1. Decrease muscle tension in the neck and face to allow for proper nerve function.
2. Decrease sinus congestion and improve breathing.
3. Cleanse digestive system and liver to eliminate bad bacteria and toxins.
4. Improve lymph flow through the body.
5. Improve digestion to allow proper elimination of toxins and healthy absorption of nutrients.
6. Improve posture to decrease tension on spinal cord.

Allergy Testing

The next test I recommend for your child is allergy testing. You must identify, address, and then eliminate the allergens within your child's body.

I had my first allergy testing when I was 11 because I was having so many asthma attacks. Once I had tested positive on all the skin tests they performed, the doctors concluded that I was allergic to basically everything in my environment. I also tested positive for some foods (shellfish was one). My parents had to get rid of the carpet in my room and put plastic on my bed—they were constantly running me back and forth to the hospital with asthma attacks. They almost wanted to put me in a bubble for protection.

The worst asthma attack I can remember was when I was 13 years old. I had lasagna and a big bowl of ice cream at an Italian restaurant. About 15 minutes after eating, my lungs completely shut down; once again, my parents had to rush me to the ER. Ten years ago, I found out when I eliminated dairy from my diet, my breathing got better because I wasn't so congested. Then three years ago, I eliminated gluten from my diet due to finding out about my thyroid autoimmune disease, and my overall health improved. I also lost 60 pounds.

There are a variety of allergy tests to determine potential IgE-, IgA-, and IgG-related immune responses. Positive reactions to skin or blood allergy testing can also be a helpful way to discover a particular allergen. In the case of food allergies or sensitivities, the best way to confirm a reaction for your child is to do an elimination test and then re-challenge the food you suspect to be a problem.

Food Allergies and Sensitivities

All our new clients do our Wellness Kids program, which includes a specific elimination diet for 30 days, and everyone notices a huge difference when we eliminate the most common food sensitivities. If your child is not improving within two weeks, I suggest getting a food allergy test done. Food sensitivities may be caused by many factors, among them stress, infections, overeating, artificial preservatives, additives, molds, pesticides, antibiotics, and environmental pollutants. Unidentified food sensitivities can then contribute to chronic health conditions, including irritable bowel syndrome, small intestine bacteria overgrowth (SIBO), rheumatoid arthritis, headaches, autism, ADD/ADHD, eczema, chronic ear infections, gut absorption issues, insomnia, and many others. When we reintroduce a specific food, we do so one at a time (and at least three days apart) so that we can check for any kind of reaction. The reaction can be a skin rash, bloating, joint pain, and/or just feeling tired again. Have your child listen to their body—it will speak to them.

Common Allergenic Foods

Common allergenic foods that we do not want your child to consume during the elimination challenge are the following:

Corn

Corn is a heavily subsidized crop, and it's used in every product you can imagine. The SAD (Standard American Diet) is riddled with corn—in fact, 75% of your grocery store is *corn*. This is also the food that is most often genetically modified.

Eggs

Another overconsumed and highly processed product is eggs. Unless chickens are raised organically or as pastured/free-range chickens, they are fed antibiotics and kept in cages with no sunlight or ability to roam. They're also often fed soy and corn, which are common allergens. (Even organically raised chickens are often fed soy and corn.) Eggs are a common food allergen that most people are unaware of.

Shellfish

Shrimp, lobsters, crabs, and oysters cause the greatest number of food reactions. This allergy usually develops later in life, although

I was highly allergic to shellfish as a child. I still avoid it for the most part, but now that my immune system is stronger, I can eat shellfish without having any reaction.

Soy

Soy is used in nearly every processed product and even some organic/natural ones. It is difficult to get rid of this substance, but we ask you to reduce consumption of it as much as you can. Hidden/different names that soy uses: monodiglycerides, soya/soja, yuba, TSF or TSP (textured soy protein), TVP (textured vegetable protein), lecithin, and MSG. Soy is also genetically modified on a regular basis.

Tomatoes

We consume tomatoes regularly and all throughout the year, and we can wind up highly sensitive to it because of those years of overuse. This nightshade vegetable can create a lot of inflammation in our body.

Peanuts

Peanuts are found in a large number of frequently eaten foods. Nearly 100 Americans die a year from this allergy. Peanuts are also usually riddled with pesticides unless purchased organic. (Alternatives to peanut butter include almond butter and sunflower butter.)

Dairy

Processed dairy products (including milk and cheese) are mucus-forming and create inflammation throughout our body. As many as 50 million Americans are lactose-intolerant. Dairy is not necessary for human diets. Traces of DDT and toxic "banned" pesticides are *still* found in conventional milk. (Alternatives include almond milk and coconut milk.)

Wheat/Gluten

Common examples of gluten-containing grains are wheat, barley, rye, and oats. Like dairy and soy, gluten is in a myriad of foods, so always read labels and beware of aliases such as flour, spelt, cake flour, couscous, matzoh, matzah, kamut, and graham.

Blood Panel Testing

Now that you have had your child's thermography and food allergy tests done, it's very important for your child to get a comprehensive blood panel done.

In a comprehensive blood panel, I am looking for blood sugar issues, anemia, gastro/intestinal dysfunction, immune imbalances, inflammation, thyroid function associated with antibodies, vitamin D levels, mineral deficiencies, and liver and kidney function markers.

Urine and Hair Testing

Also, it is good to test for environmental chemicals in your child's body through urine or hair testing. Each type of testing has its limitations, but I find hair to be helpful. In the hair analysis, I am looking for toxic elements and essential elements. Whenever we address toxic metals, I see huge turnarounds in children's overall health. There is no better feeling to me than helping a developing child who is struggling with the effects of toxicity.

Stool Analysis

Getting your child's gut healed is a must when healing the immune system and brain—remember, 80% of your immune system is in your digestive system. That's why I spend the majority of my time focusing on healing your child's gut. A comprehensive stool analysis is vital because it helps assess digestive and absorptive functions, detect pathogens and/or parasites, and identify specific bacteria and yeast.

Subluxation and Upper Cervical Care

Another test we do in our office to determine if your child has a subluxation is a neurological exam and specific upper cervical X-rays if necessary. What is a subluxation and what is upper cervical care? Upper cervical care is a branch of chiropractic practice and is defined as the discovery and removal of the vertebral subluxation, which is interference that is taking place in your central nervous system (CNS). It is important to recognize that our CNS is the master controller of our entire body and that it directly correlates to our ability to function and exist. If your child's body is not getting the information it needs from their brain, their body will be at dis-ease, as I like to say. (I prefer to pronounce it as "dis"-"ease" rather than "disease." The idea is to *not* create health issues by just focusing on an ailment—the term "dis-ease" means a lack of ease or harmony within the overall body.)

Maybe you are wondering where a subluxation comes from. It is the direct result of everything your child does—whether they're positive or negative, lifestyle stresses result in nerve interference, which then needs to be addressed. For example, during the holiday season, many kids tend to consume a substantial amount of unhealthy food and sugar and spend more time with family (which some would consider stressful). What I have seen is that after the holiday season, kids typically get sick. That's often caused by a subluxation. The unhealthy food and sugar and increased family time represent lifestyle stresses (even if the latter is considered positive) because our body is extremely sensitive to external factors. Therefore, upper cervical chiropractic care needs to be an essential component of your child's life. Not only that, it's something we encourage your entire family to consider doing.

Upper cervical doctors are different than other chiropractors. We use specific, laser-aligned X-rays to help us determine how to correct your child's spine. To perform the right correction to the upper spine and head, X-rays need to be performed to measure and examine your child's unique anatomy.

Another tool I use is thermography, which I explained earlier. I use paraspinal thermography (heat reading) to establish the pattern the nervous system is making and then monitor the readings during each visit. The kids call it the tingle machine!! I believe your child should hold their own spinal correction for as long as possible, so I only correct your child's spine when the thermography objectively indicates that a correction is needed. If I find that I am correcting your child's spine every time I see them, that is a sign that your child's lifestyle is creating an imbalance; at that point, I will need to review some lifestyle changes with you and your child so that your child can heal. Healing starts when your child is holding their correction and their brain-to-body communication is 100% flowing.

As an upper cervical doctor, I don't snap, twist, or pop the upper spine—instead, I use a gentle realignment procedure to bring the head and neck into better balance. To help your child feel less stressed at my office, your child goes to our nice resting suite to relax after they receive an upper cervical correction. This suite is cell-phone-free, and it's a place where I play relaxing music to help their body relax. I have encouraging words on the walls to help my kid clients think positive thoughts as they BREATHE!!

At my office, we take the upper cervical chiropractic lifestyle to a level where it becomes *real* for your child. Not only do we offer upper cervical correction, we consider your child's entire body and your lifestyle choices when developing customized protocols for your child to follow. These protocols combine individualized programs with tips on fitness, nutrition, and stress relief.

Children who are suffering from diseases like allergies, asthma, headaches, etc., are often living subluxated, but when we provide these children with upper cervical correction, we can remove the interference. Often, the symptoms associated with these conditions then dissipate. In addition, for children who are under regular upper cervical chiropractic care, we can actually prevent these situations from impeding upon their lives.

Adrenal Function Testing

One way to monitor your child's stress is to check their adrenal function. Adrenal saliva testing, the iris contraction test, and postural low blood pressure testing are ways to monitor your child's adrenal function.

Adrenal Saliva Testing

These days, it is generally accepted that saliva cortisol testing is the most accurate test—it gives a better estimate of the cortisol levels within your cells, and that's where the hormone reactions are actually taking place.

Here's another important thing to know about cortisol testing: taking a single measurement (or even a 24-hour average) is not enough. The best cortisol tests take four individual samples at various points of the day and then map your cortisol levels over the course of a 24-hour cycle. Our cortisol levels vary dramatically, starting at high levels when we wake up, then tapering off until they reach their lowest point late at night. This usually represents something like an 80% drop, which is perfectly normal. However, every test I have analyzed has indicated some kind of malfunction to this rhythm. Yes, even kids have stress, and it causes major disturbances within their bodies, too.

Iris Contraction Test

First described by Dr. Arroyo in 1924, this test measures the contraction of the iris in response to repeated exposure to light in a dark space. In those with weakened adrenal function, the theory goes that the iris will be unable to maintain its contraction for long.

To conduct the test, sit in a darkened room in front of a mirror with your child. Take a flashlight and shine it across your child's eye, from one side to the other. In a hypo ("low") adrenal state, their pupils will not be able to hold on to a contraction for more than 2 minutes and thus will begin to dilate despite light repeatedly shining on it. (Our irises should contract to pinpoints when exposed to bright light.) In those with healthy adrenals, the contraction should last much longer.

Postural Low Blood Pressure Testing

When we stand up, those of us who are in good health experience an almost immediate rise in blood pressure. In contrast, adrenal fatigue sufferers will see no change in their blood pressure; they may even experience a slight fall. In very general terms, a larger drop in blood pressure signifies a more severe case of adrenal fatigue, meaning that your child's body is crashed out.

This is a very simple test to do at home: just use a regular blood pressure monitor to check your child's blood pressure while lying down, then have your child stand up and check the pressure again.

EGG Brain Mapping

Lastly, I recommend getting an EGG brain map done. Brain mapping is a process that allows us to visualize inside your child's brain and very clearly identify the irregular brain waves that cause neurological issues. From that brain map, a report is generated for each child showing the areas of dysfunction and the protocols recommended to address each of them.

A brain map is performed by placing a shower cap-like cap on the head and then using software to capture the electrical impulses in the brain. This method is known as an electroencephalogram (EEG). All the child feels is some cooling gel on their head. The results show brain wave patterns in various parts of their brain. The process takes about 15 minutes, after which point the data is converted into a visual brain map report showing the results in a clear and concise format that can be easily understood. I am looking at the major functions of the brain, such as its cognitive, emotional, memory processing, and executive functions (and more). I do this by analyzing each lobe of the brain (frontal, parietal, central, temporal, and occipital) for each type of brain wave (Delta, Theta, Alpha, and Beta).

Your child's brain produces four primary types of brain waves: beta, alpha, theta, and delta. Beta is primarily active during your child's awake state, which is most of your child's day. Alpha deals with their subconscious and is dominant during relaxed states when their eyes are closed but they are not asleep. Theta is present briefly during the periods before your child falls asleep and before they fully wake up. Delta is primarily active when your child is asleep.

All of these brain waves are equally important to your child's health; not surprisingly, neurological disorders can be attributed to specific brain waves. For example, when a child has brain irregularities caused by a head injury, their brain may have too much frontal theta or delta being produced when they are supposed to be awake and alert. By retraining the abnormal patterns in the affected areas, symptoms can be improved or eliminated.

Upper Cervical Care Therapy

Now that you know what tests to do for your child, let's move on to the therapies I recommend. First and foremost, I recommend upper cervical care for many reasons. Upper cervical doctors concentrate on the brain-to-body balance. They use a very gentle technique that is very effective on small children. Because the correction is so close to the brainstem, the upper cervical doctor expects immediate changes in the overall function of the body. Here is a story about a girl named Jamie that may help you to understand what I'm talking about. (Her mom wrote down the story.)

Jamie fell inside the house when she was taking off her shoes on March 14, 2008. At the time, she was 8½ years old and in the 2nd grade. She had a 14-month-long migraine due to the concussion she had in conjunction with the fall.

Before meeting Dr. Corinne Weaver, Jamie tried adult migraine meds, in-hospital IV treatment, physical therapy, massages, swimming, and running. None of these treatments worked.

Ever since her fall, Jamie had had a daily headache and her eyes were always dilated. When Dr. Weaver took spinal X-rays of Jamie, the results made Jamie's mom think of a question mark.

After Jamie's first upper cervical correction, her headache went away and her eyes were no longer dilated.

After a few months of care, another round of X-rays were taken. Her entire spine was back in alignment without having made any adjustment to the rest of her back.

When Jamie got braces in January of 2010, the headaches and dilated eyes came back. After a quick appointment with Dr. Weaver and an orthodontic adjustment to take the pressure off her teeth, Jamie's headaches were gone and her eyes went back to normal. Then Jamie sustained another concussion. Dr. Weaver's office was the first place her mom brought her, because she had learned from the last experience and didn't want Jaime to suffer again like she had before.

Earlier, I mentioned how eyes can become dilated when the sympathetic nervous system is activated. In this case, Jamie's concussion had caused inflammation in her brain and vagus nerve, which led to Jamie's headaches and dilated pupils.

Jamie got under upper cervical care at my office and saw improvements after her first correction. She was glad someone had told her to come to my office and her mom had listened.

Massage Therapy

I also recommend neuromuscular massage to help balance the nervous system with the muscular system. This type of massage helps release tension so your children can hold their upper cervical corrections longer. Massage is also known to decrease pain and depression. As a result, children can use fewer meds. Yay—no more meds!!

Music Therapy

Music therapy can also be very healing to your child's body. We play healing music in our office; I also recommend certain tones to listen to for healing when you're at home with your children. There is quite a lot of research on the topic of music and healing! On a blog post titled "Healing Through Music" (on www.health.harvard.edu), I read that music improves outcomes when invasive medical procedures are necessary and that music has also reduced the use of opioid painkillers. The blog also stated that music therapy can restore lost speech from a stroke or traumatic brain injury, reduce the side effects of cancer therapy, aid in pain relief, and improve quality of life for dementia patients. Music touches people's hearts and can renew us by making us feel relaxed. When I do neurofeedback with kids, I have them listen to healing and calming music.

Breathing Therapy

Physical breathing is being aware of each breath through your nose. To maintain the proper level of carbon dioxide in our lungs, we need to control the rate and depth of each breath. I will discuss this more in Chapter 5.

Aromatherapy

Aromatherapy uses essential oils from plants to improve health and reduce stress within your child's body. Aromatherapy has been around for thousands of years. I have been using them for about 12 years; they've become part of my daily routine. I use them for stress relief, to lift my mood, to increase my memory and energy, for pain relief, for digestive issues, as a sleep aid, and lastly to boost my immune system. I will go over my favorite oils in Chapter 6.

Exercise Therapy

Exercise is also a key therapy. Much like a healthy diet, moving can benefit your child's body-to-brain connections and can shield your child from stress. Exercising increases brain chemicals like endorphins and GABA, and moving your body increases the blood flow to your brain. Just like your muscles, your brain cells need to be a little bit stressed to grow. When you move, put some thought into how you're moving, and you will enhance your awareness and ability to concentrate. Another idea is a trampoline—we have a trampoline at my house, and my kids love it! Here are some added benefits of trampoline training.

Trampoline Brain Training

- Reduces stress
- Stimulates flow of the lymphatic system
- Stimulates every cell in the body with every bounce
- Cleanses body and brain cells

The kids and I love to jump and play games! Having a trampoline is very beneficial for kids with sensory issues.

Fun Trampoline Games

- **Bum Wars:** Whoever can jump, sit, and land back on their feet the most without falling wins. Being physically heavier helps, so I usually win this one if I am playing.
- **Poison Balls:** Put some balls on the trampoline (we use old tennis balls), pretend that the balls are poison, and run and jump while trying to avoid them. If someone is touched by the ball, they are out. The last person standing wins.
- **Memory:** Because the brain is being stimulated with each bounce, kids can remember facts easier. For example, you could yell out a state and have your child yell the capitol back to you.
- **Hot Stuff:** We have a stuffed animal on the trampoline with us, and he/she is "hot." (Kind of like Hot Potato.) We throw the animal back and forth and play music. When the music stops, the player who is holding the stuffed animal is out.

Have fun testing out these games! If you come up with others, please do share them with me.

Laughter Therapy

Laughter is medicine for the soul, and it's free!! I find it to be the best medicine. My funny dad made me laugh a lot during my childhood and my mom had the loudest laugh I've ever heard; I can still hear her laugh today if I tune in to my old memories. My husband is also a comedian in my eyes, and I love the fact we can laugh together as a family.

Laughter increases circulation and improves the delivery of oxygen and nutrients to all parts of the body. If you suspect you might be suffering from laughter deprivation, look for ways to laugh more! We love to watch Jim Gaffigan and his family jokes. Families that laugh together, stay together. Also, make sure you can laugh at yourself, too!!

Prayer as Therapy

Prayer has been shown to have a profound effect on our health, too. Developing a relationship with God can affect everything, and surrounding yourself with a community of faith can provide even more support when your children need it the most. The members of a faith community can strengthen your resolve to heal and can link their prayers to yours. There is healing power in prayer! I believe God answered my prayer when I asked Him "What do you want me to do in life?" If we just make the time to listen, He will answer us. I love listening to Joel Osteen's podcast for encouragement.

Nutrition Therapy

Nutritional support is needed to help sick kids get well. After I review all diagnostic testing, I create a customized nutritional plan based on your child's individual needs. (You can see an example of a plan on my website.) I will go over the most common supplements I recommend in Chapter 7.

Neurofeedback Therapy

Last but not least is neurofeedback therapy. Neurofeedback is a process of training brain waves into regaining their healthy patterns using modern technology. This noninvasive and drug-free approach uses brain imaging technology to record brain wave activity and identify unhealthy brain wave patterns. Once irregular patterns have been identified, they can be corrected using guided audio and visual feedback. This amazing technology has proven itself effective over decades of research. Both studies and real-world applications show that neurofeedback works with conditions such as depression, anxiety, ADHD, fibromyalgia, migraines, and a host of other disorders.

Each neurofeedback session takes about 30 minutes. The number of sessions needed will depend on the individual—much like going to the gym, every person requires a different length of time to improve. It usually takes 20-40 sessions for many conditions to improve.

Neurofeedback sessions involve your child relaxing for 30 minutes while they watch a movie or listen to whatever music they choose. Electrodes are attached to your child's scalp that monitor their brain waves during the session. When irregular patterns are detected, the software triggers a response that pauses or dims the video or music. Your child's brain senses the change and subconsciously modifies itself back into a normal pattern. With repetition of this process, eventually your child's brain learns to stay within healthy ranges on its own without neurofeedback.

Again, the results will vary from person to person. Some feel different within a couple of sessions, while people with more difficult conditions need many sessions to see any noticeable results. The type of neurofeedback training we offer in our office is permanent. Neurofeedback helps to improve functions such as concentration, short-term memory, speech, motor skills, sleep, energy levels, and emotional balance.

Long-term follow-ups have been done on many patients. Dr. Joel Lubar at the University of Tennessee has followed ADD clients who've sustained their improvements from neurofeedback for 10-20 years. Research published on epilepsy patients 12 months after brain training shows that the effects of neurofeedback on epilepsy usually stick. Owners of the Clear Mind System (which is what I use in my office) have reported no relapses from patients even after 10 years.

Neurofeedback has been around for decades. To date there are thousands of studies, with more being published every day.

There is also a Clear Mind take-home focus unit which never becomes outdated because it can be continually updated—each take-home unit is completely programmable to suit your child's specific health needs. What's even better, this unit can be continually adapted as your child attains new levels of well-being. As your child improves, the system changes with your child!

The take-home unit brings light-and-sound technology to your child's fingertips. With my guidance, your child can have a personalized system designed to optimize their health care program. Remember, the brain emits different types of waves. Through light-and-sound technology, during a 30-minute session, your child's brain wave frequency changes speed and morphs into a healthier and more normal pattern. Your child's body-mind function becomes enhanced.

Regular use of the take-home unit combined with your doctor's care means that your child can achieve their long-term health goals.

I would like to share another story with you, this time about a high school student who was not able to focus well, especially when it came to reading. He would space out a lot and have thoughts he couldn't process or let go of. He also had a lot of trouble getting good sleep. When I first started working with him, he was very skeptical that brain training therapy would work. But as he and his family started seeing positive changes, he was excited to come to his sessions!

He started seeing these changes within the first couple of weeks of therapy. (His family started noticing differences before he did, actually.) He is now able to go to sleep and stay asleep most of the night. He can focus on his homework better, be less anxious, and control his running thoughts—now he can relax and only have one thought at a time.

This young man had been struggling with his attention issues and anxiety for a very long time. He had tried all of the therapies I talked about previously, but he never managed to fully improve with regards to his two main symptoms. He needed neurofeedback to help heal his brain. Since he was already doing the other therapies (and eating very healthy foods, too), he saw quick results.

Neurofeedback Therapy helpful when dealing with Anger

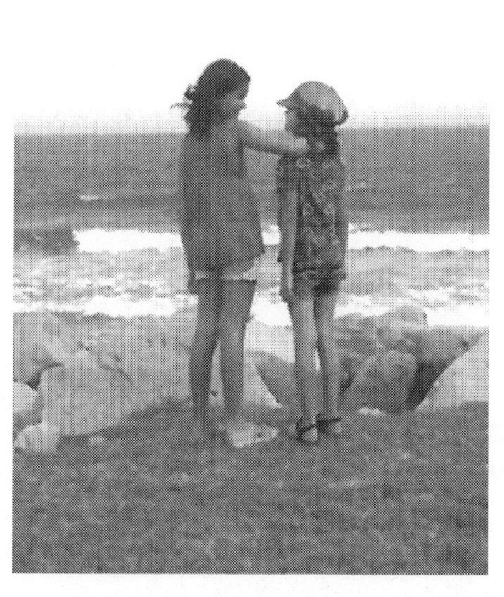

One day, my daughter Cora came home wanting to eat tacos because it was Taco Tuesday. My son did not want tacos, so I decided to fix chili soup with beans. Well, Cora was upset that tacos were not being served on Taco Tuesday. She yelled at me and said, “I hate you, mom!” I just looked at her and didn’t say anything—instead, I just smiled. Then she remembered that I had taught her to jump on the trampoline when she gets angry, so she decided to go jump on the trampoline. She was able to jump out all her feelings on the trampoline and then came to me afterward and apologized.

I am very excited to see that Cora's brain is healing! Even though she gets angry at times, she's able to do things to overcome her anger and then express love. Her anger does not last long, and she is able to control it so much better now than before she did neurofeedback.

The Importance of Routines

Why do kids need routines? Routines give them a sense of security and help them develop self-discipline. One of the biggest causes of family stress is simply too much to do in a brief period of time. Sit down with your family and make decisions about the traditions that are most important to all of you. For example, my son wanted to play basketball in our driveway versus playing on a team at school.

As examples, I'll tell you about my kids' routines. With small kids, our routines sometimes do get a little off, but keeping the same routines does help reduce stress and chaos. For one thing, I find that worship music helps us stay relaxed and stay in a mood of praise and gratitude. Here is an example of how to establish a routine. I encourage you as parents to use this as a master example to help create your own schedule.

My kid's morning routine	My kid's night routine
1. Put on worship music, wake up your child, and have them do wall angels or 10 jumping jacks to get their blood pumping while laughing. 2. Teach them to make up their bed—doing that makes their room feel cleaner. 3. Eat a healthy breakfast, drink a full glass of alkaline water and take supplements, and apply essential oils. 4. Get dressed and brush teeth with Doterra's On Guard toothpaste or my homemade one. 5. Apply natural lotion. 6. Brush and fix hair. 7. Put your smile on—you're never fully dressed without a smile!	1. Eat a healthy organic dinner with the family and talk about each other's days. 2. Start a to-do list for the next day. 3. Lay out clothes for tomorrow. 4. Pack healthy lunches. 5. Take night supplements and herbs like fish oil and probiotics. 6. Take a shower and wash hair with chemical-free shampoo. 7. Brush teeth. 8. Put lavender essential oil in diffuser in bedroom and apply to neck/lymph nodes. 9. Read the Bible, pray, and write in gratitude journal. 10. Do physical breathing exercises and give mom and dad kisses!!

What action steps are you going to take today for your child?

Action Items:

Decide what tests you should do for your child.

1) ______________________________

____

____

2) ____

____

____

Pick one or two simple habits you can incorporate into your child's daily life to improve the state of inflammation in their body.

1) ____

____

____

2) ____

____

____

Chapter 5

R-ELAX AND RELEASE

The third letter of my S-T-R-E-S-S system is "R" for *R-elax and release.* Let's relax and take the time to release our stresses and just breathe!!

Have you ever just sat and listened to your child breathe? Did you know that breath channels energy and vitality? Have you ever noticed that when your child is stressed or anxious or sick, their breathing is shallow? Have you noticed that your child's breathing is deep and full when they are free of stress and anxiety?

Most people have heard of the "fight or flight" response, which is how the body reacts when we're stressed or scared. Many people, however, have never heard of the "rest and digest" response. The parasympathetic system (where the vagus nerve is located) activates these more relaxed functions of the body, the functions that help maintain a healthy, long-term balance in life.

The central nervous system and the parasympathetic system are both part of a larger system named the autonomic nervous system, which controls and influences the way that our internal organs function. While we think that we just have just one nervous system, actually, we have several.

If your child is suffering from a lot of stress, chances are that their "fight or flight" response has been activated far too often in the past. These kinds of stressors prompt the body to release enormous amounts of stress hormones like cortisol. Over the long term, chronically elevated stress levels lead to body organs becoming depleted of the materials they need to produce the key hormones and neurotransmitters that are necessary for healthy brain function.

The Autonomic Nervous System

The sympathetic nervous system, or what generates the "fight or flight" response, prepares our body for emergency reactions. All of the organs that are involved in getting ready for a physical challenge ("fight") or preparing for a retreat ("flight") are activated through this system. The parasympathetic nervous system ("rest and digest") helps produce a state of equilibrium or balance in the body. Both are part of the greater autonomic nervous system, which is responsible for involuntary and reflexive functions in the body.

The Sympathetic Nervous System

The sympathetic nervous system is faster-acting than the parasympathetic system—it moves along very short, fast neurons. The sympathetic nervous system activates part of the adrenal gland, which then releases hormones into the bloodstream. These hormones in turn activate the target muscles and glands, causing the body to speed up and become very tense as well as more alert and ready. Functions that are not immediately essential (like the immune and digestive systems) are shut down to some degree when the body is in this state.

Your body goes through several changes when the sympathetic nervous system is activated:

- Heart rate increases
- Bronchial tubes in your lungs dilate
- Pupils dilate

- Muscles contract
- Saliva production is reduced
- Stomach stops many of its digestive functions
- More glycogen is converted to glucose

These changes are designed to make you readier to fight or run from a physical (and sometimes not-so-physical) threat. Nonessential systems like digestion and immunity are given much lower priority; at the same time, more energy is made available to your muscles, and your heart rate increases. This is what happens when we are faced with a stressor.

The Parasympathetic Nervous System

The parasympathetic nervous system (or the "rest and digest" system) is a much slower system that moves along longer pathways. The parasympathetic system is responsible for controlling homeostasis, or the balance and maintenance of the body's systems. The parasympathetic system restores the body to a state of calmness and allows it to relax and repair itself.

The body undergoes several specific responses when the parasympathetic system is activated:

- Saliva production increases
- Digestive enzymes are released
- Heart rate drops
- Bronchial tubes in your lungs constrict
- Most of your muscles relax
- Pupils in your eyes constrict
- Urinary output increases

These changes are designed to maintain long-term health, improve digestion, conserve energy, and maintain a healthy balance within your body's various systems.

How These Systems Are Activated

The sympathetic nervous system protects us from real physical dangers (like lions, tigers, and bears, oh my!) and kicks in automatically in response to any fearful thought. This doesn't have to be an imminent physical threat—any perceived threat or stressful situation can trigger this response. For example, if your child had to speak in front of their peers, they probably would feel their heart racing and their mouth dry up. In this example, hormones released by the adrenal glands are telling the heart to speed up and the body to restrict digestive processes like saliva production. Other stressors might be things like school deadlines, waking up late and missing an activity, or having dance recitals/sport events.

Many diseases and illnesses have been shown to be the result of chronic stress: cardiovascular issues, high blood pressure, and immune system suppression are classic examples. Other conditions include constipation and digestive issues, cold sores, jitteriness, sweats, and anxiety. In the long term, more advanced adrenal fatigue can lead to symptoms like chronically low energy levels, respiratory problems, and much more.

The less time we spend in sympathetic response mode, the better. Although it makes us alert and better able to respond to the challenges ahead, after a while, it takes a huge toll on our bodies and can lead to adrenal burnout, making us crash out. Anything we can do to keep our kids feel safe and stay in the "rest and digest" mode as much as possible is worth the effort—their long-term health may depend on it!

To activate the parasympathetic nervous system, learn what truly makes your child feel relaxed. Have fun with them, let them engage in a hobby, hang out with friends, exercise, or even just get them out into nature and listening to the birds sing. Whatever it is, pay close attention to you and your child's feelings and thoughts (and then try to recreate those special moments so you can both relive them when the kids are all grown and out of the house).

We are all under some level of chronic stress these days. By learning how to activate your child's parasympathetic nervous system and reduce the effects of your child's sympathetic nervous system, you can reduce the stress on their heart, digestive system, immune system, and more. This will not only make your child a happier person, it will also help your child avoid many diseases and conditions associated with chronic stress and adrenal fatigue. If you can help your child become more conscious of the way their body reacts to stress, those efforts will pay enormous dividends in the future.

We know beyond any doubt that stress can be detrimental to children's health, and we also know that record numbers of people now report feeling stressed. It may be challenging to deal with, but stress is something we need to combat if our children are to lead healthy, happy lives.

Knowing how to relax and neutralize stress is one of the keys to being happy and living a long, healthy life.

So, how can your child get rid of stress in their life? Here is the secret: they can't! Stress is a part of life. But what we *can* do is address some issues and help your child handle stress better. Here's the game plan.

Helpful Tips for Dealing with Stress

Just as we can exercise some control over the sympathetic nervous system (just thinking of a public speaking engagement can trigger a response for many people), we can also activate the parasympathetic nervous system. Simply reading a joke book does the trick for some kids. For others, soaking in a hot bath with Epsom salt and lavender, getting a massage, or petting a dog or a cat are good relaxation strategies. My kids love doing yoga—did you know now there's baby yoga?

Half of the space in my office is designed to help your child relax: after your child receives an upper cervical correction at my office, they go back into my resting suite and lay down to deep-breathe while we play soothing music and diffuse essential oils. Our kids love that time—they use it to relax and allow their bodies to heal.

Breathing

Breathing is one of those automatic body functions that is easily taken for granted, but our breathing patterns are actually quite revealing—when we need to feel centered, we stop and breathe deeply, for example. Unfortunately, however, shallow breathing is a way of life for many kids. It causes a limited amount of oxygen to reach the bloodstream and can result in fatigue, gas, insomnia, muscle cramps, and feelings of anxiety and panic.

When we encourage our kids to breathe deeply, fully, and completely, we counteract the stresses of modern life and calm their mind and spirit. Breathing not only oxygenates the body's 100 trillion cells, it also releases carbon dioxide waste material from each cell.

Smooth, deep diaphragmatic breathing improves blood circulation, gently massages internal organs, promotes elimination of carbon dioxide, strengthens the heart and lungs, and promotes deeper sleep patterns.

The next time you find your kid in a stressful situation, have them sit back and allow some time to just breathe. I love the song "Just Breathe" by Jonny Diaz!! It is my theme song. Listen to it today if you have not heard it. It talks about having a crazy busy life and only having time for yourself…but then you realize there has to be something else to this crazy life. The singer reminds you to "Rest at Jesus' feet and just breathe." This is what I am telling you now!! Help your child clear their mind and evaluate their body responses. Allow them to take the time to relax and just breathe.

When I was a kid, I had to learn how to relax whenever I would start to have an asthma attack, which is the scariest thing on earth. It's like being a fish out of water or like having thousands of bricks stacked onto your chest.

If you've been lucky enough to never have an asthma attack, think of this as an analogy—as kids, mom always used to tell us to chew our food slowly, right? Ever wondered why? Because chewing slowly promotes proper digestion by allowing the digestive enzymes in the saliva to start breaking down your food at the beginning of the digestive cycle. Similarly, proper breathing can also affect our biology.

When I was pregnant, I also learned the Bradley method of childbirth and delivered my kids naturally at home. Yes, that is right—I had all three of my kids at home with no drugs!! I was able to use the Bradley technique to avoid much of the pain and create more bonding memories with my precious babies. The Bradley method of childbirth is giving birth naturally while you're coached by a partner. My husband Scott was a pro after Noah (our first child) was born! The Bradley method helped me relax through my breathing so that I could reduce my pain and have a memorable, un-medicated birth.

Physical Breathing

Everything we do affects our biology, be it eating, exercising, sleeping…or breathing.

Physical breathing involves being actively aware of each breath! It also involves having a good standing "deep breathing" posture. Good posture strengthens the abdominal organs and increases circulation to them. We have to encourage our kids to have good posture.

What's the big deal about breathing through your nose and not your mouth? Basically, it comes down to how our breathing affects the carbon dioxide (CO2) levels in our lungs and blood. It has very little to do with oxygen levels.

Proper CO2 levels (which regulate the healthy—and narrow—pH range of the blood) allow for the adequate release of oxygen to our tissues and brain. Throughout our lives, many of us have been given the vague impression that CO2 is bad for us. Quite the contrary! Without CO2, we wouldn't get the oxygen we need. Proper CO2 levels are what trigger our red blood cells to release the oxygen they carry.

Most of the CO2 that we use does not come from the air we breathe in—rather, our own bodies manufacture CO2 as a byproduct of our natural body processes. If our children aren't breathing correctly, then they are also not producing the proper levels of CO2 in their bodies that they critically need.

Consider an unopened can of soda. It's full of fizz. We've all experienced what happens when you leave an open can out for a while: when you come back later, the drink is flat. It has lost its fizz.

What's in a can of soda? Water, salt, sugar, coloring, and CO2 (hence the term "carbonated beverage"). Interestingly, blood contains the same main ingredients: water, salt, sugar, coloring (from the hemoglobin in our red blood cells), and CO2. What would happen if our blood lost its fizz?

The lungs store CO2. The brain is set to trigger breathing through the diaphragm as long as there are adequate carbon dioxide levels in the lungs—you will achieve and maintain the proper level of carbon dioxide if you breathe functionally. If carbon dioxide levels fall below a certain level of pressure, however, we start to experience imbalances that then become symptoms.

Functional adult breathing is 8-10 breaths per minute at rest, all taken in and out through the nose and not through the mouth. Functional breathing is also driven by the diaphragm, not by the upper chest. Most importantly, breathing should be silent—if breathing can be heard, it's not functional.

Knowing how many breaths your child takes while at rest can help you determine if they are breathing normally. A child who has a fever or who feels anxious breathes faster than normal.

- A newborn under 6 months of age takes 30-60 breaths per minute.
- A 6-month-old to 12-month-old child takes 24-30 breaths per minute.
- A child who is 1 to 5 years old takes 20-30 breaths per minute.
- A child who is 6 to 12 years old takes 12-20 breaths per minute.

Advantages of Nasal Breathing

Noses are made for breathing! Nasal breathing (as opposed to mouth breathing) increases circulation, boosts blood oxygen and carbon dioxide levels, slows the breathing rate, and improves overall lung volumes (7).

Noses have a four-stage initial filtration system:

1. The hair filters out the particles in the air
2. The mucous contains an enzyme that kills viruses and bacteria
3. The sinuses warm and condition the air
4. Nitric oxide is produced and improves lung function

Before the air enters the lungs, it goes through two final filters that are outside of the nose: the adenoids and the tonsils.

This multi-part system is important because the lungs are very sensitive and therefore respond better to air that has gone through the four filtration stages of the nose rather than only going through the mouth. "The internal nose not only provides around 90% of the respiratory system air-conditioning requirement, but also recovers around 33% of exhaled heat and moisture (8)."

Close your mouth!

In a child who breathes heavily through an uncovered mouth, we often see three immediate problems:

1. Lower CO2 in the lungs
2. Lower CO2 in the blood
3. Restricted O2 flow to the brain and other tissues

Low CO^2 Levels Are a Problem

Low CO2 levels cause the blood pH to rise toward its alkaline limit, at which point an alert is sent to the brain. We need to control the rate and depth at which we breathe by means of physical breathing. This is done using the diaphragm. If we don't use the diaphragm as the primary muscle of breathing, we will have problems maintaining the correct carbon dioxide level within our lungs—when we breathe through our mouths, we use our upper chest to breathe and we don't use the diaphragm correctly.

By directly controlling our diaphragm with physical breathing, the brain tries to limit the amount of CO2 that we lose. In short, if your child breathes correctly, they will restore balance to their body and will be able to change the way they feel.

What to do now? Ask your child to close their mouth, open their nose, and breathe in health! In Chapter 8, I go over some physical breathing exercises.

Accumulated Stress

Here's the secret: it is not calendar years that are stealing your child's quality of life, it's built-up damage from stress, errant thinking, and lack of physical movement.

We can all relate to this—everything starts when we're kids, but we don't notice it. Stress and the repercussions of stress just keep building up. Then suddenly, one day you "wake up" and begin to see and feel the results.

While you can't change your calendar age, you *can* resist or even reverse years of stress damage if you're not too late. The sooner you start, the better your results will be! This is why I love starting with kids—if I can start with them, I can really change our world's health. It's all about learning science-based secrets for ageless living and shattering the perpetual myths that cloud your vision.

It's gut-wrenching for me to see a new patient walk into my wellness clinic who is too far gone for me to help them reverse their pain and ravaged health. In some cases, sadly, too much damage has been done for too long. Now you know why I love seeing parents act to improve their kids' health early on! A lot of times, the parents don't want their kids to suffer like they did.

Seeing a mom or dad fight for their kid's health makes me want to be the best doctor I can be. It takes a mom and or dad to *believe* that their child can get well before health can happen. Parents who fight for their children and who are willing to work hard with our program and with their children on a daily basis see results. Don't give up! Listen and act. Are you ready to take action *today*?

Go to www.physicalbreathing.com for more information.

Action Item:

Pick one or two simple habits you can incorporate into your child's daily life to improve their state of relaxation.

1) ____

____

____

2) ____

____

____

Chapter 6

E-SSENTIAL OILS

The fourth letter of my S-T-R-E-S-S system is "E" for *E-ssential oils.*

Essential oils are part of my morning and night routines. Most people wake up in the morning and use heavily (and artificially) scented shampoos and soaps. They put aluminum-containing deodorant under their arms, which clogs up the lymphatic system. They use dryer sheets with artificial scents to make their clothes smell good. All of these chemicals are toxic and are closing up our pores and not allowing our bodies to breathe properly. Long-term exposure to chemicals found in hygiene products, cosmetics, sunblocks, fragrances, detergents, and everyday household cleaners causes toxin overload. This stresses the liver and adrenals and causes the body to have disease.

Instead of breathing in all of those chemicals and toxins, breathe in essential oils and herbs. Be cautious when supplementing with these for the first time! Use one product at a time and see how your child responds, then gradually build up the dosage as they get healthier.

In addition to their intrinsic benefits to plants (the compounds in the oils constitute the plant's immune system) and being beautifully fragrant to people, essential oils have been used throughout history in many cultures for their medicinal and therapeutic benefits. Numerous plants have been identified as having antimicrobial, antiviral, or antifungal properties (9,10,11). Modern scientific studies and overall trends towards more holistic approaches to wellness are driving a revival of essential oil health applications (and new discoveries, too!).

Essential oils are used to promote a wide range of emotional and physical wellness aspects. Depending on user experience and desired benefit, essential oils can be used a single oil at a time or in complex blends. They are usually administered by one of three methods: diffused aromatically, applied topically, or taken internally as dietary supplements. I love putting a drop behind my ears and rubbing it on the back of my skull and on my lymph nodes in the morning and at night. We are forever diffusing my office with therapeutic aromas using a variety of essential oils. Everyone enjoys the wonderful smells we create! Using essential oils can be both profoundly simple and life-changing at the same time.

Essential oils are plant compounds taken from the roots, stems, barks, and leaves. I have over 50 oils in in my house, but here are the top ten you can use to improve your overall health and mood.

Top 10 Essential Oils

1. **Peppermint** oil was the first essential oil I used (over 15 years ago). I commonly use it now to treat runny noses, digestion issues, cramps, and tension headaches. It is very invigorating and antiviral. I also use it in my morning routine to wake me and my kids up.
2. **Lavender** oil is great for stress relief, healing burns and boo-boos, and improving sleep. It also protects the brain and has been used to treat concussions.
3. **Orange** oil is my favorite smell, especially Doterra's wild orange oil. It is a mood lifter; I love to use it in my lotions and room fresheners. It can change a moody kid into a happy kid just with its smell.

4. **Frankincense** is a very powerful, effective oil and can cross over the blood-brain barrier. It helps relieve chronic stress and anxiety. Using it can boost your child's immune system and reduce pain and inflammation.
5. **Atlas cedarwood** oil is a very cool name, I think, because I love the atlas human bone. Cedars were the trees most often mentioned in the Bible as a symbol and source of protection. I find this oil to be helpful for kids who have trouble focusing—this oil has a very warm tone and helps improve their mood. It also strengthens their immune system when your kid is under stress.
6. **Vetiver** oil was found to be the most beneficial oil to help ADHD. That study was performed by Dr. Terry Friedmann, MD, and Dennis Eggett from Bringham Young University. They found that inhaling vetiver oil improved focus in children with ADHD by 32%. This oil calms and balances the nervous system while stimulating the circulatory system.
7. **Lemon** oil is a great cleansing agent. I also use it to help my allergies (along with lavender and peppermint). It improves lymph drainage and also cleanses the body.
8. **Clove** oil is the oil I use most often in my house for its anti-everything properties. For example, it is antibacterial, antiparasitic, and antifungal, and it offers antioxidant protection. I love it in our toothpaste!
9. **Cinnamon** oil stops the growth of bacteria and fungi in the body and may help increase brain function. It also reduces blood sugar levels in diabetics and helps lower cholesterol. When it comes to antioxidants that help fight disease, cinnamon ranks at the top of my list. Every morning I put cinnamon in my apple cider vinegar drink. Not only does it taste fantastic, it can relax the tracheal muscles in the lungs and help me breathe. I love this in our toothpaste, too.
10. **Rosemary** oil can also be used to help with brain function and memory. It increases alertness (unlike lavender, which calms you).

Using a combination of these in a diffuser will freshen up the air in your house and help everyone breathe better; these oils will also improve your child's mood. Be careful when using these oils, though, because they are very powerful. Start slow and build up! As I said before, I started with only peppermint oil and over the course of 12 years have expanded that to 50 oils.

It's easy to clean with essential oils—they are safe and effective. I enjoy making my own cleaners so that I can reduce the amount of harmful toxins in my home.

For more information on these oils and helpful tips, you can go to: my LIVE event called No More Meds or watch my webinar on www.drcorinne.tv. I love to educate parents so that kids can stay healthy all year long. Together we can transform pediatric healthcare and get 1 million kids off of meds that may not need! Join the No More Meds Movement with me and get your child healthy!

Chapter 7

S-UPPLEMENTS AND HERBS

The fifth letter of my S-T-R-E-S-S system is "S" for *S-upplements and herbs.* When I was a kid and my Uncle John would come into town, he would use some wonderful herbs to make me a tea. I would put a kitchen towel over my head and breathe in the tea's steam for about 30 minutes, then drink the tea. It felt so refreshing to be able to breathe so well!

Just as I did when I was a kid, all children respond to gentle herbs. Using herbs for health reasons can be very beneficial, but knowing *how* to use herbs safely is very important. Coming to our live workshops can help you be more confident about using herbs for your family's needs. Find out when our next Live workshop is on www.physicalbreathing.com.

There are thousands of useful herbs on this planet, but I use my top ten herbs daily. It was hard to pick the top ten because God's plants are so useful in so many ways!

Have you ever tried any of these herbs? If not, what are you waiting for? You will be amazed. If you do purchase any of the below herbs, make sure you are getting them in their purest form.

Top 10 Herbs and Spices

1. **Turmeric (curcumin)** is a spice that has compounds called curcuminoids, the most important of which is curcumin. Curcumin is the main active ingredient in turmeric. It is one of the most powerful natural anti-inflammatory herbs in the world (12). I have this in my shake every morning. It's deeply yellowish-orange and stains everything it touches, so don't get it on your clothes, towels, or light-colored kitchen utensils.
2. **Ginger** is in the same family as turmeric. Ginger is the spice of my life! I love it in everything. It makes our smoothies and meals taste so good and also aids in relieving nausea. (It was very helpful with my morning sickness days during my pregnancies [13].) It is also very anti-inflammatory (14), so next time you are making a smoothie, just throw in a little fresh ginger root! I also like making ginger tea: peel the fresh root and dice a one-inch slice into 15-20 pieces, then steep in hot water for about 30 minutes before enjoying. I like adding some lemon or lime and a dash of honey for a little extra zing.
3. **Plant digestive enzymes,** specifically the enzyme in pineapple, which is bromelain. It is a great digestive aid, it supports immune function, and it reduces inflammation. Bromelain is very helpful for people who have chronic sinus issues; it has a long history of use as a remedy for sinusitis. Recent clinical trials have found positive benefits for children with sinusitis who take bromelain (15,16).

   Because plant digestive enzymes help break down food so that you can better absorb the nutrients, it's best to take the enzymes before you eat. Veggies provide these essential digestive enzymes, so you will be less likely to react to them. There are also great green (fruit and veggie) drinks that you can consume daily to get all the enzymes you need. It is clear from numerous studies that children and adults who consume a variety of fruits and veggies have a lower risk of allergies and associated asthma.

4. **Garlic** may be stronger than an apple when it comes to keeping the doctor away—it's antiviral, antibacterial, and antifungal (17). Also, mixing garlic oil with eucalyptus and/or melaleuca essential oils can be useful for treating ear infections. You can make your own garlic oil mixture by warming up some olive oil (about 4 ounces if you're making a big batch) on low heat and adding chopped garlic (about 4-5 cloves). Cook on low heat for 30 minutes. Strain the oil through a cheesecloth, then add 20 drops of eucalyptus and 10 drops of melaleuca. Store in an amber bottle. Using an eye dropper, place 2 drops in the ear and then massage behind the infected ear every hour or as needed (usually 2-3 days). For additional soothing, fill a sock with salt and mullein flower oil, then warm it before placing it around the ear. Having a great upper cervical correction also helps clear up an ear infection.
5. **Elderberry** is great to use for upper respiratory issues because it is known to relax respiratory muscles. I love Natranix from Orthomolecular—it contains echinacea, thyme, and sage. Every time I travel, this item goes into my bag for extra immune support.
6. **Chamomile** is one of the best all-around herbs for kids—it calms the nervous systems of children suffering from anxiety and is great for colicky babies with tummy aches.
7. **Rose hips** contain a lot of vitamin C, so they offer the same benefits that vitamin C does, plus rose hips also contain trace minerals. Making a rose hip tincture can be a fun thing to do with the kids. Visit our website for a video on how to do this.
8. **Echinacea** is an immune-enhancing herb and is only used when a child is fighting an illness like a cold or the flu. Orthomolecular makes a product called Imu-max; it tastes great.
9. **Lemon balm** is another mild nerve sedative. I love using it to de-stress. (It goes well with chamomile!) Lemon balm can also help alleviate fussiness.
10. **Goldenseal** came in handy after I gave birth to my first child—my midwife told me to apply it to my child's belly but-

ton to help prevent infection where the umbilical cord was. It was amazing: within five days, the rest of the cord fell off, and his belly button was normal. I have found this herb to be helpful for minor skin wounds.

Top 11 Supplements

1. **Psyllium seed/husk** for fiber. Why do I say we need to get more fiber? Because the number-one complaint I hear in my office is gut issues. Kids today are not getting the right amount of fiber! I strive for at least 30 grams a day. According the Institute of Medicine, women need 25 grams of fiber a day and men need 38 grams per day. Previously, I stated that children need 19 to 31 grams per day depending on their age, so stating "around 30" is safe.

   When I am analyzing my kids' diet sheets before they start with me, I calculate that the typical kid gets about 15 grams of fiber a day (or less) in their diet. Fiber is a great way to help your child's body remove toxins. Of course, take plenty of water with psyllium, because it expands like gel in the intestines. Psyllium is very high in fiber and cleans the colon. It also reduces bloating and gas and helps lower cholesterol to a healthier level. Fiber is considered to be vital for eliminating toxins from the body, limiting the stress those toxins place upon the immune system, and helping us breathe better. I love a product called Ready! Set! Go! from Orthomolecular. It also contains prunes and figs for added benefits.

2. **Vitamin D** is very crucial for immune health (18). Vitamin D comes from the sun, so we need to go outside to take in all the sunshine. If you can, go outside now with your child and get some warm sunshine. Usually just 10 minutes a day in the midday sun is all you need. (Let that little light of your child *shine*!!) Some other ways to get vitamin D are cod liver oil and certain fish.

Vitamin D can also reduce your risk of getting autoimmune disease. When I found out I had antibodies in my thyroid and that my vitamin D levels were low, I immediately started taking more vitamin D. That blood test I did three years ago was a wake-up call for me! I encourage you to get your child's vitamin D level checked. I check this when I do a comprehensive blood panel at my office.

As for me, I no longer have symptoms of Hashimoto's (fatigue, overweight, constipated, sensitivity to cold, skin dryness, puffy eyes), which is an autoimmune disease of the thyroid, and I lost 60 pounds over the course of two years. After I got my energy back, the first thing that came to my mind was, "I need to write a book."

3. **Fish oil** with high amounts of EPA/DHA and GLA. These fatty acids reduce the overall inflammatory burden and improve brain function. A three-year study concluded that if a child received fish oil supplements between the ages of 6 months and 3 years, they had a reduced rate of allergy-related coughs (19). Fish oils also promote normal growth of blood vessels and help repair nerves. Think of the Tin Man in the Wizard of Oz—grab the oil can and squirt it on your joints to keep them from squeaking! (By that, I mean take fish oil internally before going to bed.) I always tell this to my patients so that they understand the concept of how important fish oil is. If you are allergic to fish, take flax or chia seed oil instead.
4. **Probiotics** are the good guys (i.e., the good bacteria) that help combat the effects of the harmful guys (i.e., bad bacteria, yeast, and fungus). As we are being born, we pick up microbes from our mom as we pass through her vaginal canal. Unfortunately, babies born by Cesarean section don't pass through the birth canal and therefore miss out on the benefits of picking up their mom's protective microbes. Researchers believe that the epidemic-level increases in asthma, allergies, type 1 diabetes, celiac disease, and obesity are related to disturbanc-

es in the microbiome, which is fueled in part by microbes—microbes help train the immune system (20). That is why I called my favorite probiotic The Good Guys, it can be found on my website.

As a society, we have overused antibiotics and have messed up our guts. I have heard multiple doctors say that we need to be on a probiotic for an entire year to recover from one dosage of antibiotics. Harmful bacterial organisms are so smart and have become so antibiotic-resistant! But do not let them outsmart you. Remember, the herbs and supplements I've mentioned can help fight off those bad guys, and if you do wind up needing antibiotics, you can use those same herbs and supplements to help your gut rebound.

Multiple strains of probiotics are constantly being discovered, which is why I am constantly changing the probiotics my family takes. It is good practice to start your child on one and then change it every time you buy another bottle. Even though my kids have never had any antibiotics and were born vaginally, I still give them probiotics daily. Several strains of probiotics have also been shown to limit some allergy symptoms (21).

You can also eat and drink probiotic-rich, fermented foods like sauerkraut and kombucha. I love making kombucha—my favorite one is made with green tea, ginger, lemon or lime, and strawberries. Yum, yum, good!! To see how to make kombucha, check out the kombucha video on our YouTube channel; we also have information on our Facebook page. ("Like" us to continue getting helpful tips: www.facebook.com/getwellnc.)

5. **Zinc lozenges** are able to directly inhibit the rhinovirus, which can affect our breathing. Zinc is a vital trace mineral involved in over 300 different enzymatic reactions in the human body. Because zinc enhances our immune system, if we don't have enough of it in our system, we are more susceptible to infections (22). The body can't store zinc, so we need to get

it through our diet or as a supplement. How can you check to see if you are deficient? This is the test we do in our office. Metagenics makes a product called Zinc Tally. It is a simple screening method for evaluating zinc status. By placing two teaspoons of Zinc Tally in your child's mouth, a lack of taste or a delayed taste perception suggests a possible zinc insufficiency. If that happens, we recommend that kids add zinc to their diet and then we check on them again a month later. If your kid's gut is inflamed or if they are having stomach pains I use my product called Strengthen Your Gut which contains zinc, vitamin A, L-glutamine, N-Acetyl-D-Glucosamine, Licorice root, and Aloe Vera. This product was designed to promote the health and barrier function of the gut lining.

6. **Magnesium** is a wonderful mineral that helps relax the bronchial tubes and the smooth muscle of the esophagus. I recommend using a product called Reacted Magnesium from Orthomolecular. It is a powder that dissolves very well. This product has worked well for my patients with asthma, ADHD, insomnia, and autism. It calms the nerves down and helps them relax so they can breathe better. Another great product I use is Cerenity PM by Orthomolecular (this also includes some B vitamins).
7. **Monolaurin** is found in coconut oil and is similar to other monoglycerides that are found in human breast milk. (As we know, a mother's milk is the best food for her baby!) Monolaurin destroys protective viral envelopes and kills viruses (23,24). It also fights off bad guys like harmful bacteria, yeast, fungi, and protozoa. I have been using a product called Lauricidin for over 12 years—it is my go-to when my family is feeling a little off. You can order it at http://My.Lauricidin.com/DrCorinneWeaver.
8. **Vitamin E** has been found to reduce the risk of wheezing and eczema in children at age two (25). It also helps reduce the free radical damage incurred during the body's inflammatory response.

9. **Vitamin C** helps repair and regenerate tissues. My family takes a good amount every day to support healthy immune function. Vitamin C is very safe to take and can be very effective in helping lessen the duration and symptoms of a common cold. We use my Super Power C formula to keep us running with Super Power!!
10. **N-acetyl cystenine (NAC)** is an antioxidant that increases glutathione levels and thins bronchial mucus, plus it helps liquefy sinus mucous and removes the bad guys from the body. It also helps with pain levels. Yay!! Recent data also suggests NAC inhibits the function of eosinophils, which are immune cells known to be active in allergy-induced asthma. NAC also inhibits the immune-recruiting chemokines expressed by smooth muscle cells of the human airway (26,27). My kids and I love my Just Breathe (adult formula) and my Just Breathe Jr. (kid formula) product. It contains vitamin C, quercetin dihydrate, stinging nettles leaf, bromelain, and NAC. This is a great combination if your child struggles with allergies and you want a natural de-histamine to help them get though that season.
11. **B Vitamins!** I also have to throw in B vitamins like B12, B6, and B2. B vitamins are vital for the brain. In addition, B6 and B12, are critical for proper methylation which is vital for supporting mental health as well as immune and nerve cell function. When stress levels are elevated, additional intake of B vitamins is often needed.

Choosing my top supplements and herbs was tough, but I want you to get the most from your money when you are buying products. I would like to say you can get all the nutrients you need from your diet but let's face it our diets are not perfect and it's hard to get all the nutrients we need from the food we eat daily to achieve optimal body function and wellness all the time. *If you would like to learn more or order my supplements you can at www.DrCorinneWeaver.com.*

In summary: the only way to know what you need and how much you need in terms of nutrients is to get tested.

Are you being tested properly? I test my patients and give them what they need based on the results, which is why I am able to treat many childhood health disorders. When it comes to your child's health, search out a doctor who cares and wants you to succeed in your child's health journey.

Your child's brain health can improve if you maintain a clean environment at home, reduce your child's stress levels, eat as many unprocessed, whole foods as possible, and use nutritional supplementation and antioxidant-rich herbs.

Action Item:

Which essential oils, supplements, or herbs will you incorporate into your child's daily life to improve their immune system and brain?

1) ______________________________

____

____

2) ______________________________

____

____

Chapter 8

S-LEEP

The final letter of my S-T-R-E-S-S system is "S" for *S-leep*. Our kids must sleep!

Getting extra sleep and relaxing are critical healing components for your child—babies, children, and teens need significantly more sleep than adults do to support their brains and physical development. Millions of people throughout the world don't get enough rest and sleep. This is a major health problem! Kids are tired all the time. According to the National Sleep Foundation, newborns need 14-17 hours of sleep each day/night, babies between the ages of 4 and 11 months need 12-15 hours, toddlers need 11-14 hours, preschoolers need 10-13 hours, school-aged kids need 9-11 hours, and teenagers need 8-10 hours. I also recommended having your kids go to bed before 8 PM every night. Having a consistent and soothing wind-down routine (as previously mentioned) can help your kids get better sleep. I've heard from multiple doctors that the hours before midnight are the most valuable for sleeping and healing because of the energy of the earth and sun. Have you ever stayed up past 1 AM and then regained energy and couldn't get back to sleep? I have done that multiple times.

The best and safest sleeping position for your child is in on their back with pillows under their knees and a small neck pillow. If possible, have them sleep with their legs and arms straight and slightly out to the sides. Also, make sure their pillow is not so big that it cuts off some of their air supply. I have had to correct many kids' spines because of the way they twist and turn in their sleep. Sleep position is crucial to keeping the right posture!

Lastly, make sure you clean the pillowcases often; otherwise, your child will be breathing in lots of dust and bacteria (it comes off their head and then sticks on their pillow). If your child is still a baby, the best way for them to sleep is on their back and with nothing in their crib.

Relaxing When Awake: Breathing from the Belly

According to posture expert Dr. Steven Weiniger, "Diaphragmatic breathing is also called breathing from the belly. A good, deep, cleansing breath should originate from the belly, not the chest."

How do you know if your child is breathing from their belly? Place one of your child's hands and one of your hands on their belly and the other on their chest. Tell them to take a deep breath. The hand on their belly should rise as their diaphragm fills with air, while the hand on their chest should stay still. If you feel the hand on their chest rise with each breath, your child will to work towards making belly breathing the normal way they breathe! Chest breathing means shallow breathing, and that leads to stress, shortness of breath, dizziness, and higher levels of anxiety.

Here are some wonderful physical breathing techniques for you to do with your kids. Enjoy doing your physical breathing!!

Physical Breathing Techniques

Belly Breathing

The first thing your child (and perhaps you) will need to learn is what's called "belly breathing." This is the most basic breathing method we can do anytime; therefore, it is the one you should master before trying out any of the others. It's very simple—it just requires a few steps.

1. Have your child sit or lay down comfortably, depending on their personal preference.
2. Have them place one of their hands on their stomach, just below their ribcage. Place the second hand on their chest.
3. Tell them to breathe in deeply through their nostrils while thinking positive, healing thoughts and letting their first hand be pushed out by their stomach. Their chest should not move.
4. Tell them to breathe out through their nose, expelling all of their negative thoughts. Gently press on the hand that's on their stomach, helping them press out their breath.
5. Slowly repeat 3 to 10 times.

They should begin to feel relaxed as soon as they have repeated this belly breathing exercise two or three times, but keep going for as long as you feel they need to. After they have mastered this breathing exercise, there are four additional methods for them to try (they range in difficulty).

4-7-8 Breathing

The method called 4-7-8 breathing also requires your child to be sitting down or lying comfortably. Here are the steps:

1. Your child should be in the same position as they were for the belly breathing exercise, with one hand on their stomach and one on their chest.
2. Breathe in slowly but deeply through the nose. Take 4 seconds to breathe in, feeling the stomach move during the process.

3. Hold the breath for 7 seconds.
4. Breathe out through the nose as silently as possible, taking 8 seconds. Once your child has reached the count of 8, they should have emptied their lungs of air.
5. Repeat as many times as needed, making sure to stick to the 4-7-8 pattern.

Roll Breathing

If you are looking for a breathing exercise your child can do comfortably while sitting down, try the "roll breathing" method. Its aim is not just to relax, but also to encourage the full use of your child's lung capacity. Your child might want to lie down during their very first time, but after that, they should find it just as easy to sit while completing this exercise. Follow these steps:

1. Again, start with the belly breathing position: one hand on the stomach and the other on the chest. Your child's hands should move as they inhale and exhale.
2. Take a deep breath from the lower lungs; breathe slowly, ensuring that the chest hand doesn't move. Use the nose to breathe in and out.
3. Repeat these deep breaths 8 times. On the ninth repetition, once your child has filled the lower lungs, they should take a breath to move their chest up. This will fill their entire lung capacity.
4. Gently exhale through the nose, being sure to empty the lungs. While exhaling, make a small whooshing noise. Both of your child's hands will move down as both the stomach and chest fall.
5. Practice this method for 4 to 5 minutes. When exhaling, your child should be able to feel a tangible difference in their stress levels.

Morning Breathing Routine

While the above three exercises can be done whenever necessary, the next method is called "morning breathing." As its name suggests, this should be practiced once your child has woken up. Morning breathing aims to relax their muscles after a good night's sleep and help them minimize tension for the remainder of the day. Here are the steps:

1. Have your child stand up straight. With slightly bent knees, bend the torso forward from the waist. Both arms should be limply hanging close to the floor.
2. Take in a breath slowly while returning to the original standing position. Your child should look like an inflatable Gumby balloon while doing this, with their head being the last thing to straighten up.
3. Exhale again, again bending forward while exhaling. Stand up straight after finishing, stretching the muscles as required.

Night Breathing Routine

The deep-muscle relaxation technique is the most time-consuming, but it can also be the most rewarding for your child's body. This works best when combined with belly breathing; it is a wonderful way to attain full relaxation. Doing this technique will exercise each major muscle in turn (although have your child pay the most attention to any muscles that are causing discomfort or aching). To start, have your child lie down in a comfortable position and focus on belly breathing, closing their eyes if need be. While playing soothing music, have them do the following:

- To relax their face, have them knit their eyebrows together, then release.

- To relax their neck, have them tilt their head down towards their neck and push their chin to their chest, then release.
- To relax their shoulders, have them make a shrugging motion, then release and roll.
- To relax their arms, have them push both arms away from their torso, stretch them out, and then relax them by their side.
- To relax their legs, have them point their toes as much as they will stretch, then relax.

All of these stretches should be done while doing the belly breathing we covered earlier. Breathe long and deep and take time with each stretch. My kids and I enjoy doing this with soothing ocean sounds in the background.

Action Items:

Imagine yourself walking on the beach when you come across an unusual bottle. You pick it up and rub it. Suddenly, a genie appears and grants you three wishes.

What would your three wishes be for your child?

1) ____

2) ____

3) ____

Ideally, all of us want to be happy, so I ask you this: what makes you and your child happy?

____

____

Not that I have already obtained all this, or have already arrived at my goal, but I press on to take hold of that for which Christ Jesus took hold of me. Phil. 3:12

Chapter 9

LET'S FIGHT FOR OUR CHILDREN!

I'd like to share two stories of parents fighting for their children.

Ear Infections Resolved

One child was a little girl who had chronic ear infections. In the space of five or six months, she had multiple infections and been on three rounds of antibiotics. Her doctors were talking about giving her more, but the parents didn't want their daughter to take any more antibiotics—they wanted to find a permanent solution for her ear infections. Some of their church friends had told them about having success at my office, so they thought to bring her daughter to see me.

After almost a year of wellness care at our office, she has had only a few short-lived ear infections! I taught her parents how to boost her immune system and care for minor ear infections with remedies that actually work, so she recovers much more quickly now; she's only had to go to her pediatrician for her regular wellness check. She loves getting adjusted (her parents feel like this is a permanent solution to many of the health issues people are facing). She also sleeps better for the first few days after her adjustments, and she gets over her slight colds faster than her parents do!

Seizures and Hip Dysplasia Resolved

This next story is another little girl who was having seizure-like symptoms and hip dysplasia. The seizure-like symptoms started after three months of having been in a full body cast that was meant to help her hips. Eventually, she was allowed to be in her casts for shorter and shorter periods of time, and that's when she had her first symptoms: her eyes would roll and her body would stiffen in an unusual way. Her parents went to multiple doctors who did lots of diagnostic tests that could only tell them something was wrong, but the doctors couldn't figure out what.

The parents were referred to me through some church friends who had seen positive changes in their kids' colic and sickness issues after having seen me. I was their last resort. They had never heard of a gentle chiropractor, and they definitely had never heard of infants seeing a chiropractor. Of course, the adjustments I did were anything but harsh—I used minimal force, like I was gently opening a closet door using only my fingertips. They were comfortable with what I was doing as I was adjusting her.

I also educated the parents on more than just chiropractic care—I looked at how she was fed, what she was fed, and how her digestive system was doing. I told them what they could do at home to help her heal in a more natural and holistic way.

Her parents loved that the thermography pictures were a way to see how her body was responding to care without having to subject her to radiation or make her uncomfortable the way so many other tests had. They could see from her first to her most recent thermography pictures that there had been improvements. In fact, she hasn't had any more seizure-like symptoms since they started working with me.

Staying the Same Isn't an Option

Here's something that is true for both children and adults: if we are not constantly working to improve ourselves, our bodies will not remain the same—rather, we will deteriorate as we age, even when we're still young. Simply put, if we're not going forward, then we're going backward. Staying the same just isn't an option, although many people would like to think it is. But it just isn't.

So as parents, how do we move our children forward in a positive way? How can we guarantee that the next years will bring more pleasant circumstances and rewards than the last few did? The answer is really basic and uncomplicated: although there are (uncommon) exceptions, the choices we make in life determine life's outcomes. We reap what we sow.

Creating Better Habits

Start making better choices and forming better habits for your child one day at a time. Remember to always consider the long-term implications, not just the immediate gratification of what you're doing (and what your child is doing). Remember: we form habits every day.

Periodically, all of us have had to deal with bad habits. It seems that once we acquire them, they take up shop and permanently move into our subconscious mind. We know that bad habits lead to no good, yet we continue to allow them to rule over our God-given decision-making abilities. Why is this so?

Habits are formed in our minds. Just as a stream of running water cuts pathways into the earth, our habits shape neurological pathways within our nervous systems. Once these paths have formed, it's easier to follow the learned behavior than to change it. The good news is that all habits can be changed the same way they were created: one day at a time. It takes 4 to 6 weeks for these neural paths to form; not surprisingly, it takes the same amount of time to revise or interrupt them.

Can you take 6 weeks out of your approximately 4,160 weeks of life to break your child's bad habits? Yes, you can...*if* you know how to replace bad habits with good habits that lead to good results. Keep in mind that anyone is more likely to continue doing something if the outcome brings pleasure. That's doubly true if you're simultaneously removing pain.

You must adopt one important behavior if you want to achieve continued success in letting go of nasty habits: don't focus on getting rid of them! Instead, focus on encouraging **positive behaviors** and help your child make transformations slowly.

Pause for a moment and breathe in deeply with your child. Do this seven times. Yes, take this time right now and breathe. First, take a deep breath and feel your chest inflate with positive energy and refreshing oxygen. Hold this breath for a couple of moments while you both reflect on the things you are grateful for, then exhale and expel your negative thoughts, diseases, and addictions while your child does the same. Now repeat six more times and enjoy this moment in time together. Share what you're grateful for.

Here's another tip for transforming negativity into positivity: if a goal is important to you, share it with one or two of your close, trusted friends, friends who have supported your past dreams and goals. Such encouragement can also help.

The Breath of Freedom!

As your child starts to heal, you begin to feel a sense of freedom. It's really quite beautiful to feel that you're actually in control of your child's future—it's like waking up on a bright, fresh spring morning after a good night's rest! When you finally replace those negative habits with positive ones, nothing will keep your child from seizing and taking advantage of a wonderful life.

Aside from the obvious health benefits of cultivating good habits, what else might you have been missing out on by not refocusing and moving forward? A positive self-image for your child, perhaps? With improved self-image comes self-respect and discipline. With self-respect and discipline comes the desire to take on new challenges in life. As your child takes on new challenges, they will gain confidence.

Along with your child gaining confidence, you'll want to foster your child's ability to benefit others with their good habits. Positive thoughts and behaviors toward family and friends lead to others step out of their comfort zones and take control of their lives, too (as well as supporting your child's efforts). It's amazing how all these benefits accrue and follow on the heels of each other just by getting your child started on the path to a positive self-image!

Finding Time

If you're like most other people, though, you might consider it problematic to find the time in your child's hectic schedule to change their behaviors. But here's a little secret: time is always a problem (real or imagined) no matter who you are or what you do for a living!

Lack of time is the flimsiest of all excuses, but it's the easiest and most convenient one to use. Then again, many people find time to take care of themselves and exercise while working 40 hours per week. Others who work two jobs and 70 hours per week also find the time. In truth, there is no time to "find." There is only time to allocate. All of us allocate our time based on our chosen priorities. It boils down to making choices. Don't fool yourself with the "finding time" excuse—your child is the one who will lose. And so will you.

Putting Health First

You've heard me say that health is our most valuable asset. My family is most important to me, and my family is the reason I must make my children's health my number-one asset. Deny your child's proper care today, and you'll pay the price of your neglect tomorrow. You need to make your own health a priority, too, so that you can be there for your family.

Over the past 13 years, I've had the opportunity to work with thousands of patients and have seen countless families devastated by serious illnesses and debilitating diseases affecting their children, spouses, parents, or grandparents. Most of these conditions are brought on by inactivity and obesity and therefore can usually be avoided.

If you consider yourself a supportive parent and you want to place your loved ones above everything else (which is why you are reading this book), then you absolutely need to reorder your time priorities and prioritize caring for your child. Remember, time spent working with our program will be time well spent, because our program induces changes that will bring greater joy to your child's life as well as to your life. It's the joy of being there for the ones you love and the ones who depend on you!

If you still question your ability to move forward and make something happen, here's something to consider: celebrate the gift of your child and care for that gift wisely! Start by developing good habits and crowding out the bad ones.

Self-Care

Wellness is 95% self-care, so don't forget to take care of yourself, too! This book is for parents with sick and oversensitive kids, yes, but you as a parent need to stay healthy, too. You're always taking care of someone else—your children, your aging parents, a sick relative or friend, an out-of-work sibling. But what have you done for you lately?

While it's commendable to want to help others, charity begins at home, as they say. "At home" in this sense means taking care of you. If you don't do that, you certainly can't help anyone else, especially your child.

A holistic approach to taking care of you incorporates caring for your physical body, your emotions, your intellect, and your spiritual self.

Chapter 10

THERE IS NO PLACE LIKE HOME

Again, my goal is get your child's body to be at its optimal health so they can fulfill their God-given purpose.

I love teaching the fundamental principles of self-care to parents—that has pulled so many of my kid patients from the brink of despair. But once parents know the principles, your child is the one who must employ them in order to embrace a wellness lifestyle. Your child's level of self-education will continue to improve over time.

Remember These Simple Guidelines

Stress is a part of life. Have your child make the time to de-stress and enjoy the little things that matter. Make the time to plan ahead and define your purpose and what your child's purpose may be. Look your children deeply in the eyes and tell them how much you love them. Most of the time, we tend to concentrate on the problem, but what we need to do is concentrate on the positive energy within the child.

Have your kid stay away from these foods as much as possible: processed GMO foods, dairy, gluten, and sugar. Remember, the perimeter of a typical grocery store is filled with both the healthiest and the freshest foods! Avoiding the center aisles will save you from unhealthy foods and may also save you money thanks to your family being in better health. Perhaps skipping the traditional grocery store entirely and focusing on produce markets/greengrocers, farmer's markets, and natural co-op stores.

Eating more veggies and fruits provide higher levels of nutrition along with essential digestive enzymes and cofactors and is less likely to cause a reaction. In addition, focusing on these foods helps children eliminate or reduce their consumption of processed foods. Eat at home—there is nothing like a home-cooked meal, especially when it is prepared with love.

Search out a doctor who listens to your concerns and is willing to help find the root cause of your child's illness. Don't give up! Keep fighting for your child's health. At times remember to just breathe, relax, and release all of your negativity. Learn how to use essential oils, supplements, and herbs when needed. Come to our live workshops or webinars.

Make sure your child is getting enough sleep, because most of your child's healing happens when their eyes are closed. Remember, too, that your children have the power within themselves to heal any ailment with their BREATH!!

I want to leave you with Jessica's words. She is a patient who first came to see me in 2004.

"God led me to Dr. Corinne in October of 2004 when I was 22 years old and at the lowest point in my life. At that time, I was struggling with many health issues, including severe acid reflux, depression, anxiety, and irritable bowel syndrome. I had been struggling with these conditions for over five years (since my junior year in high school). My parents had taken me to numerous doctors and specialists, ranging from my pediatrician to specialists at Duke Hospital to a regular chiropractor. Nothing had helped, not even the surgery for acid reflux,

which was a last-resort effort. After spending my high school and college years seeing numerous doctors and undergoing multiple tests, I was truly at the end of my road. I was suicidal and just wanted the Lord to take me from this Earth.

Then I started receiving upper cervical care from Dr. Corinne. Within 18 months, I was prescription-free thanks to chiropractic care and supplements. Thankfully, ever since then, I haven't been on any prescriptions for any of the health issues I had been previously dealing with. It was a true miracle for me to no longer have any symptoms of acid reflux, depression, anxiety, or irritable bowel syndrome. Dr. Corinne was able to pinpoint my underlying issue immediately, and I haven't had any neck/back pain since then.

All of my problems started in February 1999 after I was involved in a wreck. I had X-rays at the time of the wreck, and of course the ER physician said that everything was fine—I just had whiplash and would be better in about two weeks. Just take the prescription pain pills, he said. That took care of my soreness, but all the other health issues I mentioned previously began within a month.

Fast forward to 13 years later. I still receive upper cervical care every three weeks, as do my husband, two sons, grandparents, and mother. Dr. Corinne was one of my biggest supporters through my pregnancy. I didn't have any issues at any point in time. My 13-year-old son no longer has any asthma symptoms since receiving upper cervical care, and he hasn't had a sick visit with a pediatrician in four years. My youngest son started chiropractic care immediately—within 12 hours of being born, he had his first upper cervical correction. He is now three years old and has never had a sick visit with a pediatrician. He has only been there for preventative visits. He takes supplements daily and he loves the essential oils Dr. Corinne recommends. At the first sign of any sickness, we start the essential oils, load up on supplements, and run to Dr. Corinne's office for upper cervical chiropractic care. About 99% of the time we need to be adjusted, and then we are back to par within a day or two.

I am extremely thankful that God led me to Dr. Corinne 13 years ago. I feel 100% that if He had not, I would not be where I am today. I might not even still be on this earth still striving to serve Him. Thank you, Dr. Corinne, for your wonderful care that has allowed my body to heal itself naturally without drugs. Your love, care, and commitment to my family is amazing, and we are all forever grateful. I have no idea what we would do without you and upper cervical care. You are truly a godsend. You are my 'life line.' Much love to you, and may God continue to use you to bring healing to people's lives. I look forward to many more years."

I just couldn't leave out that last testimony. As tears stream down my face, I am here to tell you I am just a plain ol' country girl whom God is using to help bring healing to others. All I wanted to do was to help one child, and today, I have helped thousands regain their health. I give all the glory to God, because He was the one who created my healing hands and opened up my heart to care for others. I hope these stories speak to your heart and help you see the LIGHT!!

If I teach you nothing else from this book, my website, and our e-mail messages, I want to teach you this Sanskrit proverb:

"For BREATH is life, and if you BREATHE well, you will live long on earth."

My wish for you is to see a miracle happen within your child.

God BLESS, and I love you all.

—Dr. Corinne Weaver, DC

REFERENCES

1. Depression and Other Common Mental Disorders: Global Health Estimates. Geneva: World Health Organization; 2017. Licence: CC BY-NC-SA 3.0 IGO.
2. www.healthline.com/health/adhd/facts-statistics-infographic
3. Light, Donald W. and Lexchin, Joel and Darrow, Jonathan J., Institutional Corruption of Pharmaceuticals and the Myth of Safe and Effective Drugs (June 1, 2013). Journal of Law, Medicine and Ethics, 2013, Vol. 14, No. 3: 590-610. Available at SSRN: https://ssrn.com/abstract=2282014
4. Blocked Atlantal Nerve Syndrome in Babies and Infants, Gutmann G, Manuelle Medizin (1987) 25:5-10
5. "A Prospective Study of Humoral Immune Response to Cow Milk Antigens in the First Year of Life" Pediatric-Allergy-Immunology, August, 1994, 5(3)
6. "Epidemiological and Immunological Aspects of Cow's Milk Protein ALLERGY and Intolerance in Infancy." Pediatric-Allergy-Immunology, August, 1994, 5(5 Suppl.)
7. Swift, Campbell, McKown 1988 Oronasal obstruction, lung volumes, and arterial oxygenation. *Lancet* 1, 73-75
8. Elad, Wolf, Keck 2008 Air-conditioning in the human nasal cavity. *Respiratory Physiology and Neurobiology* 163. 121-127
9. Rios, J.L. and Recio, M.C. Medicinal plants and antimicrobial activity. *J Ethnopharmaco. 2005;100(1-2):84.*
10. Li T. Peng T. Traditional Chinese herbal medicine as a source of molecules with antiviral activity. *Antiviral Res.* 2013 Jan;97(1):1-9.

11. Reichling J, Schnitzler P, Suschke U, Saller R. Essential oils of aromatic plants with antibacterial, antifungal, antiviral, and cytotoxic properties—an overview. *Borsch Complemented.* 2009 Apr;16(2):79-90.

12. *Chattopadhyay I, Biswas K et al. Turmeric and curcumin: Biological actions and medicinal applications. Current Science 2004;87(1):44-53*

13. *Bryer E. A literature review of the effectiveness of ginger in alleviating mild-to-moderate nausea and vomiting of pregnancy. J Midwifery Womens Health, 2005; 50(1): e1-3.*

14. *Grzanna R, Lindmark L, Frondoza CG. Ginger-an herbal medicinal product with broad anti-inflammatory actions. J Med Food. 2005;8(2):125-32.*

15. *Braun JM, Schneder B, Beuth HJ. Therapeutic use, efficiency and safety of the proteolytic pineapple enzyme Bromelain-POS in children with acute sinusitis in Germany. In Vivo. 2005 Mar-Apr;19(2):417-21.*

16. *Buttner L, Achilles N, Bohm M, Shah-Hosseini K, Mosges R. Efficacy and tolerability of bromelain in patients with chronic rhinosinusitis-a pilot study. B-ENT. 2013;9(3):217-25.*

17. *Goncagul G, Ayaz E. Antimicrobial effect of garlic (allium sativum). Recent Pat Antinfect Drug Discov. 2010 Jan;5(1):91-3.*

18. Frieri M, Valluri A. Vitamin D deficiency as a risk factor for allergic disorders and immune mechanisms. Allergy Asthma Proc. 2011 Nov-Dec;32(6):438-44

19. Peat, J.K., Mihrshahi, S.et al. Three-year outcomes of dietary fatty acid modification and house dust mite reduction in the Childhood Asthma Prevention Study. J Allergy Clin Immunol. 2004; 114 (4):807-813.

20. Jirillo E, Jirillo F, Magrone T. Healthy effects exerted by prebiotics, probiotics, and symbiotic with special reference to their impact on the immune system. Int J Vitam Nutr Res. 2012 Jun;82(3):200-8.

21. Boyle, R. J. and Tang, M.L. The role of probiotics in the management of allergic disease. Colin Exp Allergy. 2006;36(5):568-576.

22. Fraker, P.J.; King, L.E. et al. The dynamic link between the integrity of the immune system and zinc status. J Nutr. 2000;130 (5S Suppl):1399S-1406S.

23. Thormar, H.; Isaacs, C. E.; Brown, H. R.; Barshatzky, M. R.; Pessolano, T. (1987-01-01). "Inactivation of enveloped viruses and killing of cells by fatty acids and monoglycerides". Antimicrobial Agents and Chemotherapy. 31 (1): 27–31. doi:10.1128/aac.31.1.27. ISSN 0066-4804. PMC 174645. PMID 3032090.

24. Arora, Rajesh; Chawla, R.; Marwah, Rohit; Arora, P.; Sharma, R. K.; Kaushik, Vinod; Goel, R.; Kaur, A.; Silambarasan, M. (2011-01-01). "Potential of Complementary and Alternative Medicine in Preventive Management of Novel H1N1 Flu (Swine Flu) Pandemic: Thwarting Potential Disasters in the Bud". Evidence-Based Complementary and Alternative Medicine. 2011: 1–16. doi:10.1155/2011/586506. ISSN 1741-427X. PMC 2957173. PMID 20976081.

25. Litonjua, A.A. Rifas-Shiman, S. L. et al. Maternal antioxidant intake in pregnancy and wheezing illnesses in children at 2 y of age. Am J Clin Nutr. 2006; 84(4):903-911.

26. Martinez-Losa, M., J.et al Inhibitory effects of N-actylcysteine on the functional responses of human eosinophils in vitro. Colin Esp Allergy. 2007;37(5):714-722.

27. Wuyts, W. A., Vanaudenaerde, B.M. et al. N-acylcysteine reduces chemokine release via inhibition of p38 MAPK in human airway smooth muscle cells. Euro Repair J. 2003; 22(1):43-49.

ABOUT THE AUTHOR

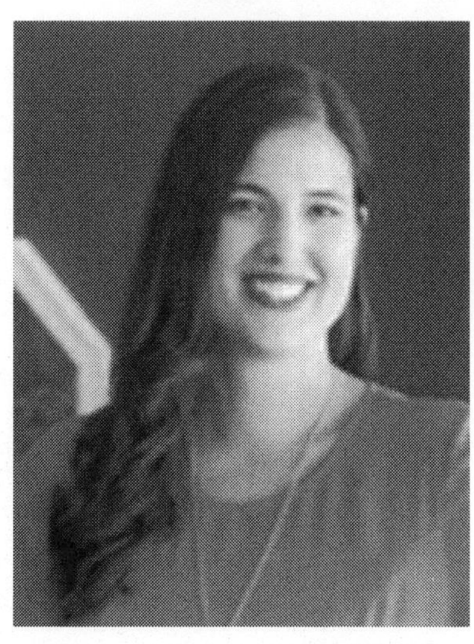

Dr. Corinne Weaver is a compassionate upper cervical chiropractor, educator, motivational speaker, mother of three, and internationally bestselling author. In 2004, she founded the Upper Cervical Wellness Center in Indian Trail, North Carolina. Over the last 13 years, she has helped thousands of clients restore their brain-to-body function. When she was 10 years old, she lost her own health as the result of a bike accident that led to having asthma and allergy issues that she thought she would always have to endure. Then, after her first upper cervical adjustment at age 21, her health began to improve thanks to upper cervical care and natural herbal remedies. This enabled her to create a drug-free wellness lifestyle for herself and her family, and she also enthusiastically discovered her calling to help children heal naturally.

Upper Cervical Wellness Center is known for finding the root cause of health concerns through lifestyle changes, diagnostic testing, nutraceutical supplementation, and correction of subluxation (as opposed to just medicating the symptoms). The practice offers cutting-edge technological care at its state-of-the-art facility, including laser-aligned upper cervical X-rays, bioimpedance analysis (measures body composition), digital thermography (locates thermal abnormalities characterized by skin inflammation), and complete nutritional blood analysis, which is focused on disease prevention.

Dr. Corinne Weaver, DC, was recently named one of Charlotte Magazine's "Top Doctors" in 2016 and is now a number-one internationally bestselling author.

THANK YOU!

Here are some goodies I want to share with you as a thank-you for reading my book.

FREE VIDEO TRAINING on 3 BIG Myths About ADD/ADHD That Are Keeping Your Children's Health Hostage. You can head on over to http://charlotteaddhelp.com/free-video/ to sign up for it.

FREE STRATEGY SESSION: Do you want to talk to me about your child's health and get my take? Great!! Go to www.drcorinne-weaver.com/index.php/apply-now/

FREE GRATITUDE JOURNAL: Having a gratitude journal can change your whole outlook on life. If you would like one, I'll send you a free gratitude journal. You will love it!! All you need to do is email me at dr@drcorinneweaver.com. We'll schedule a call to talk about your health goals, and at the end of the call, remind me to send you your gratitude journal. I'll put one in the mail to you for free.

CONTACT INFORMATION

Dr. Corinne E. Weaver, DC

14015-D East Independence Blvd.

Indian Trail, NC 28079

704-882-1488

dr@drcorinneweaver.com

Websites:

www.DrCorinneWeaver.com

www.GetWellNC.com

www.CharlotteADDhelp.com

www.DrWeaversWater.com

www.PhysicalBreathing.com

www.DrCorinne.tv

www.NoMoreMedsMovement.com